Tantric Numerology

CREATE YOUR DESTINY

Sikh Dharma Edition

Guruchander & Kirn Khalsa

© All rights reserved. No part of this work may be reproduced or transmitted in any form or by any means, electronic or mechanical, including photocopying and recording, or by any information storage or retrieval system, except as maybe expressly permitted by the 1976 Copyright Act or in writing by the publisher.

All information in this book is based on the experiences and research of the authors and others. This information is shared with the understanding that you accept responsibility for your own health and wellbeing. You have a unique body; the action of every treatment is unique. Health care is full of variables. The result of any recommendations suggested herein cannot always be anticipated and never guaranteed. The authors and publisher are not responsible for any adverse effects or consequences resulting from the use of any remedies, procedures, or preparations included in this book. Consult your inner guidance, knowledgeable friends, and trained healers in addition to the words writtenhere.

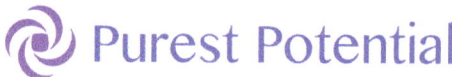

To find our more please contact us at www.purestpotential.com

Purest Potential
1505 Llano St.
Santa Fe, NM 87505
www.purestpotential.com

Editing and Formatting
Ram Krishan Singh Khalsa

Photography
Kirinsukh Westrup

© 2018 by Purest Potential

ISBN: 978-0-9903605-5-1

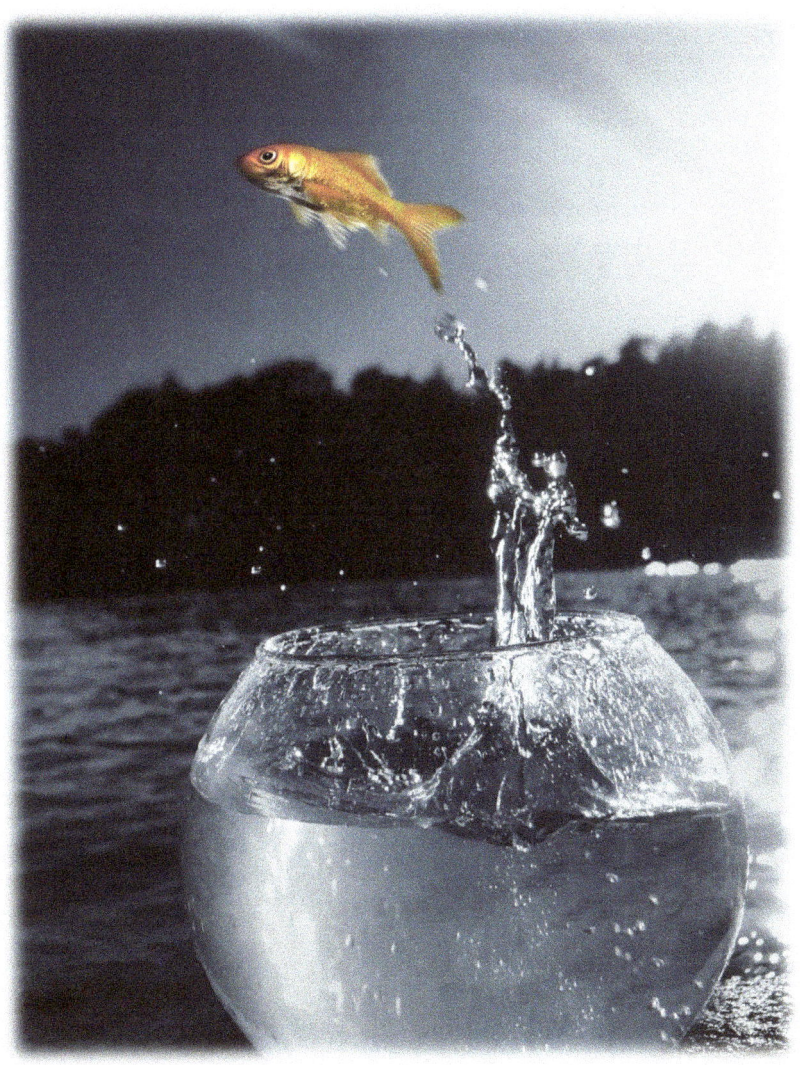

To all those who want to or have jumped out of their fish bowl to experience the potential beyond, who long to weave the polarities into an experience of integrated whole-ness, who know that when we live "in" the polarities, according to right and wrong, we lose the connection to the heart. To those who journey not only to arrive, but to do so with more of the heart and the true Self integrated *because* of the journey:

To you we dedicate our life's work with much gratitude and overflowing joy-

Kirn and Guruchander

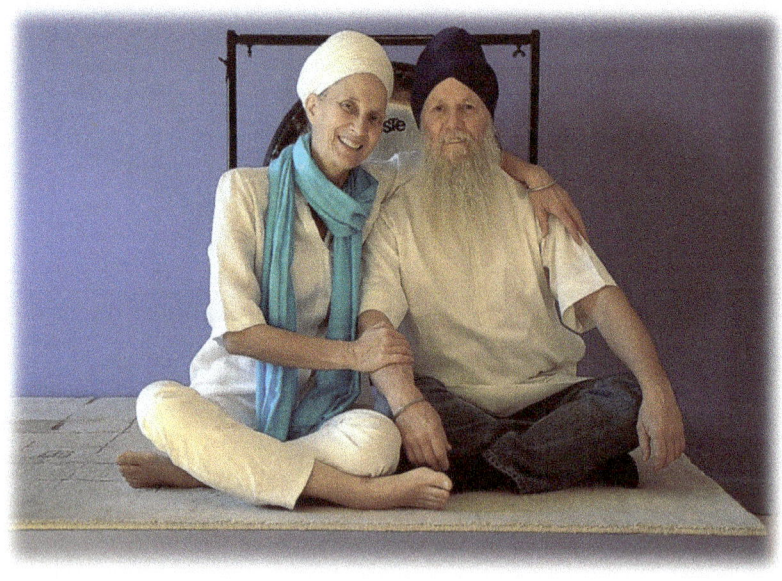

Contents

PREFACE	1
INTRODUCTION	2
THE TEN BODIES	7
First Body - Soul - Guru Nanak	8
Second Body - Negative Mind - Guru Angad	13
Third Body - Positive Mind - Guru Amar Das	18
Fourth Body - Neutral Mind - Guru Ram Das	24
Fifth Body - Physical Body - Guru Arjan	31
Sixth Body - Arc Line - Guru Hargobind	37
Seventh Body - Aura - Guru Har Rai	41
Eighth Body - Pranic Body - Guru Har Krishan	46
Ninth Body - Subtle Body - Guru Teg Bahadur	51
Tenth Body - Radiant Body - Guru Gobind Singh	58
The Eleventh Embodiment - The Siri Guru Granth Sahib	62
CREATE YOUR DESTINY WITH YOGIC NUMEROLOGY	65
YOGA PRACTICES TO CREATE YOUR DESTINY	68
Locks (Bandhas)	70
Seals (Mudras)	72
Pranayam (Subtle Breath)	74
Common Asanas	76
Mantra	78
Drishti or Eye Focus	79
Long Deep Relaxation Routine - End of Each Kriya	80
First Body	83
Second Body	87
Third Body	91
Fourth Body	94
Fifth Body	98
Sixth Body	102
The Seventh Body	105
Eighth Body	109
Ninth Body	113
Tenth Body	117
Eleventh Embodiment	121
About the Authors	**125**

Preface

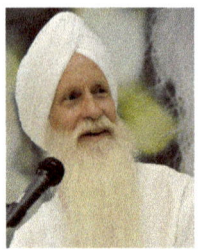

I first began learning about this system of numerology in the early 1970's. Yogi Bhajan was visiting our ashram in Eugene, Oregon and a friend and I asked him how he used numerology to determine a person's spiritual name. At the time, Yogi's answer made great sense to me in the larger and cosmic scheme of the universe. However, the next day, when I reviewed my notes and tried to make some coherent use of the information, I realized that I had no idea what it meant or how it could be used.

To my good fortune (and yours too, now that you have this book), Dr Guruchander not only took the time to explore this system with Yogi Bhajan, he also helped to expand this invaluable body of knowledge. Because of Guruchander's persistence, over the years Yogi Bhajan has continued to give more information about the ten yogic bodies, as well as examples of how to frame the numbers in ways that help you understand yourself and others.

After I took a workshop with Guruchander in Alaska, I started using numerology to counsel hundreds of people, and I have found it to be accurate, insightful, and very helpful. It is a balanced and compassionate way to help people become more conscious about themselves and others. It is also an excellent vehicle for enhancing your own intuitive interpretive abilities. I include numerology and the ten bodies as part of my yoga classes at the University of Alaska and the students thoroughly enjoy it.

The only drawback to this book is that you are not seeing and hearing Guruchander teaching in person. He is such a great teacher! His style is warm, humorous, and earthy, and he manages to convey a lot of information in a very relaxed way. He has such clarity and surety of this subject and can be so casual and entertaining at the same time. I want to thank Guruchander for his pioneering work in this fascinating area of yogic study. I know you will enjoy this book.

Nirvair Singh
December, 1992

Introduction

Tantric numerology has its roots in ancient yogic and tantric teachings, and is very applicable in today's world. It describes the ten emanations of the human psyche: the soul body, negative mind, positive mind, neutral mind, physical body, arc line, aura, pranic body, subtle body, and radiant body. As the times change so must our relationship to our self. We have moved from an agricultural to a technological culture, from the Piscean age to the age of Aquarius, and our psyche needs to expand and grow in relationship to our external world. Kundalini Yogis observe that this can be done through the awareness of the ten bodies. The knowledge of the traditional seven-chakra system was supportive to human development in the past, however, the increased pressure on our psyche requires us now to relate on more subtle levels. We need to expand the current model of awareness, and that is what this book is about.

This book is different from most numerology books. We won't be dealing with a lot of numbers or formulas. Our first book, *Numerology for Self Mastery*, presents the ten bodies in a very personal way. A good way to begin your study of the ten bodies would be to familiarize yourself with the information in the first book. It explains how to calculate the numerology hidden in the day of your birth. Your birth numbers describe your preliminary destiny in terms of the ten bodies. To expand yourself beyond those first studies of numerology and actually apply the technology to cause positive change using all ten bodies will give you the capacity to re-write your destiny. This is the aim for *Tantric Numerology*.

This second book looks at the expressions of each of the ten bodies so you can learn how to integrate and coordinate each body consciously. These bodies are the yogic representations of what the fully expressed human being feels and acts like. The practical part of it is that anyone can achieve this state of realization - it just takes applying your awareness. You don't need to belong to any organized anything to express your potential.

Knowing your personal numbers will allow you to harmonize your soul's expression. Our premise is that the soul has lessons to integrate and gifts to express this lifetime. With an awareness of your soul's journey you can manifest your unique potential. Learning how to express the full capacity of your ten bodies will give you the ability to live beyond the drama of your karma, (polarities) so you can fulfill your Purest Potential. These two books are the foundation for you to learn how to bring yourself completely present in your own life in a harmonic way.

Since the sixties, the New Age and Human Potential movements have encouraged people to become whole, to become complete. Tantric Numerology describes this expression of becoming whole and how the different parts of the psyche, the ten bodies, interrelate. This integration process is what the yogis call: "tantra". It is when we weave the polarities into something new and original. Tantra identifies the polarities and instead of fighting, analyzing, or rationalizing them, a tantra practitioner learns to use the energy, which the polarities liberate for self-actualization. In the West the word tantra is identified mainly with sex, yet this ancient practice is applicable to all aspects of living. This entire worldly existence can only manifest because of polarities; it moves because of the polarities. To express your destiny, you have to learn how to integrate polarities. This book explains that process for you.

Happiness and peace of mind are not ruled by chance, others or circumstances. We cannot control the events around us, but we can choose how we relate to those events. Instead of reacting to the polarities, we can access the ten bodies with the intention to maintain inner peace. This is where peace of mind, personal power and all the other "success" qualities people strive for come from – from you, when you harmonize your internal state.

Understanding your ten bodies can help you deal with life's ups and downs. Let's say money is tight for you and you start to feel insecure. Your insecurity could begin to manifest as lower back pain. At that point, a deeper understanding of the ten bodies would help you know that lower back pain could come from feeling insecure. It would also help you know that a strong seventh body makes you feel secure. Then you could take responsibility for your own healing and do something to strengthen your seventh body, such as a yoga set for the aura. As your aura gets stronger, you will feel more secure, and your lower back pain could be relieved as well.

As a chiropractor, I have the clinical experience of giving patients exercises to correct the aura and have seen this transform their lower back pain as well as their insecurity about prosperity. A strong aura gives an experience of security that is sustainable and constant. With this experience, you no longer block the flow of prosperity by feeling insecure from the expression of a weak aura, and like magic the money will start to flow again. Money is not really the issue; it is the experience of feeling secure. This book will reveal the deeper potential for healing and integration for each of your ten bodies.

The process of recognizing these types of clues is fully described in our third book – Purest Potential – A Yogi's guide to Brilliance.

One concern we have with current models of psychology and human potential is that they say that in order to go forward in life, you first have to heal old emotional patterns. We have found that this is not the optimal yogic approach to personal growth. Change and transformation happens in the now. Instead of looking back to heal all the things that happened to us as children, we encourage you to focus on your human experience in this moment, as it will illuminate the opportunities for transformation.

Once you understand your numerology you can focus on: "What will I feel like beyond any karmic expressions? How awesome am I going to be when all my ten bodies are balanced? How will I feel when I relate to my nobility and my radiance, versus my dramas and traumas?" We have gradually moved into a model that says there is nothing wrong, there is nothing broken, other than the inability to deepen and keep growing in awareness. The key is to not get stuck in past karmic/reactive patterns, and to live in the present, in the neutral now, and to keep deepening into the expression of your purest potential.

You know where you have karmic, self-limiting programs about life and about yourself. You will 'hear', "I am bad, I am such a loser, I am too fat, nobody appreciates me." With ten-body-awareness you can choose to change what you pay attention to and focus on your greatness, your grace, your subtlety, your compassion, and your majesty. The psychic heat you generate by focusing on your greatness will burn up all that old pain, and change the energetic patterning. So be mindful of what you energize with your thoughts because that which you "water," grows. Water the weeds and they grow, or you can water the flowers and they will grow. From this exploration of your ten bodies, you will naturally become more mindful where you put your energy (prana). You will be able to observe that your energy expands and attracts like unto like.

For the first seventeen years that I meditated, I would sit and chant and watch all my mental and emotional un-integrated issues come up, and I would continue to chant in order to eradicate all those old programs. But now when I meditate, I only focus on: "I am a yogi...I am creative... I am courageous... I am happy, bliss is here." I have code words for each of the ten bodies that I run through my mind, and when one of the code words triggers a reaction, I focus on that particular body and sit still until I can experience it as being in harmony. Once I experience harmony I chant a mantra to connect the experience to the fourth body, and then I can merge with my soul again.

Each one of the ten bodies is a very distinct space that you can fully experience in its balanced or imbalanced expression. Reading this book will help you get familiar with the "signature" and awareness of the balanced and imbalanced expression of each body. Once you recognize the balanced manifestation, it is easy to recreate it: like riding a bicycle - you don't ever forget how to ride once you've learned. You might have to sit down for a few minutes and meditate, but you can return to that optimum space by simply connecting to it, by tuning IN. The biggest gift you will receive from mastering your ten bodies is flexibility. You will be able to call on any one of your ten bodies at any time to serve you, and you will absolutely be able to come through for your Self.

Knowing your personal numerology will give you the ability to create an intentional yoga and meditation practice to strengthen your assets and integrate your challenges. When you learn how to create harmony between the ten bodies, you experience constant growth and expansion and you move towards greater and greater realization and expression of your Self. It is never static, always expanding and transforming. Tantric Numerology describes the model of the ten bodies, and the actual process for manifesting your destiny. This potential is available to any person who is willing to commit to it.

Practice with Purpose!

Supported by the following books:

> Numerology for Self Mastery
> Tantric Numerology – Create your Destiny
> Purest Potential – A Yogi's Way to Brilliance

...and now your journey begins...

With the help of our first book, Numerology for Self Mastery, we invite you to complete the following map based on your personal numerology calculations. Put your soul number by the yogi, your karma number by 'your story', your gift and destiny numbers on your 'foundational assets road', and your path number where that road leads you.

These five positions bring focus to your personal journey. From this awareness, you can design your spiritual practice. To "activate" your potential destiny we will now explore the integration of all ten bodies.

CREATING YOUR DESTINY

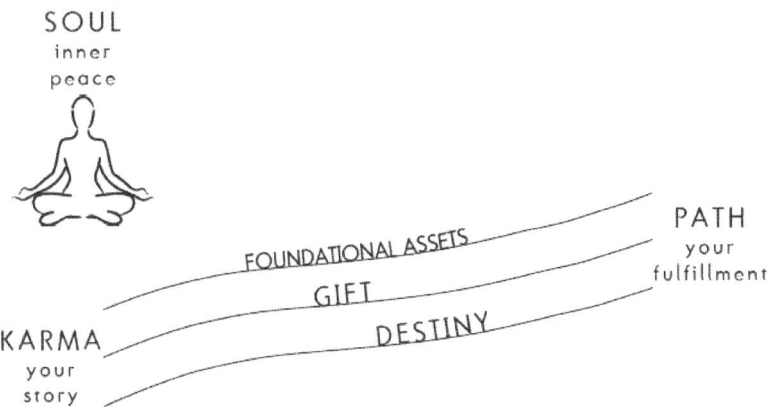

The Ten Bodies

'THE GURU IS NOT THE PERSON.
GURU IS NOT THE PERSONALITY.
GURU IS THE WORD.'

- Yogi Bhajan 1992

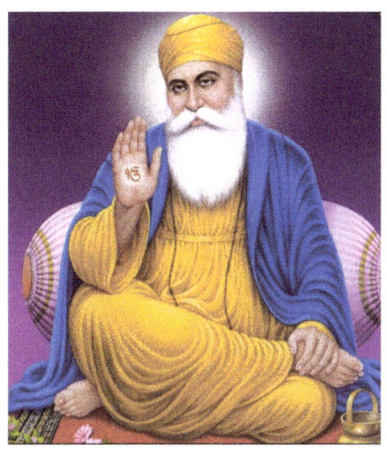

1
First Body
Archetype: Guru Nanak
The Soul Body
Creativity, Humility, Heart over Head

Guru Nanak was born in India in 1469 to Hindu parents. He was a true social reformer, and taught that all humanity is one family, that all religions are sacred, that men and women are equal, and that hard work and a householder's lifestyle are worthy paths to God. He established congregations where everyone, regardless of gender, religion, or caste, could sit together, and sing simple songs of devotion and receive inspiration.

One day Guru Nanak was herding his cows and he sat down under a tree to rest. Soon he fell into a deep meditation. His cows strayed into a nearby field and ate up all the crops. A few hours passed and Guru Nanak was abruptly awakened from his meditation by the farmer who owned the field. He was yelling and complaining that the cows had ruined his crops. Guru Nanak smiled sweetly at him and said, "My friend, the way it looks to me everything is just fine. We will go look at your crops." When they reached his fields, the farmer was amazed to see that all the crops were as they had been before, green and lush and unharmed. The cows were in a pasture nearby, grazing peacefully.

Guru Nanak embodied the spirit of love and compassion for all creatures. His example inspired many people and his teachings eventually evolved into Sikh Dharma. He became the first Guru in the lineage of Sikh Gurus in India during the sixteenth, seventeen and early eighteenth centuries.

Guru Nanak is the archetype for the first body, the soul body, the spiritual body. Spiritual disciplines teach that the soul is your basic connectedness, the voice that speaks to you, your inner best friend, the place inside that brings you peace, the touchstone of being human, that which makes you feel in harmony with the universe. The soul is the connectedness to God energy experienced within. Once you learn to experience and identify that energy within your being and to listen to that inner guidance, you automatically live in a state of harmony.

Many people use the word soul without much connection to what it means. They have little personal experience of it - they think it is outside them and that they have to go find it. The mystics' and yogis' experience is that the soul is always within and the soul is something you can consciously access. We see many people who long to find their soul through religion and yet have only been able to create an intellectual abstract relationship with the concept of their soul. Religious leaders talk about moral or ethical issues, and then the person listening evaluates him or herself in those terms and possibly resolves to change their behavior. This in the yogic world has not much to do with spirituality, with creating a connection to your soul. Spirituality is an experience of Infinity, the experience of the flow of spirit within the self.

The mystical traditions and the ancient religions were primarily concerned with this internal experience of spirit. Most religions today are far removed from creating that internal experience. I was born into a Western religious tradition that for me was very non-experiential and instead was very intellectual. It was based on what somebody else said about God, the universe and life, not me sitting down every day and having, with all of my senses, a direct experience of the relationship with Spirit.

Many were raised to believe that God is totally powerful, and that He is always watching our performance and ready to award or punish us based on that performance. As yogis we offer a different relationship with this all-powerful presence. This presence is not outside of us deciding to give or take from us. This presence is like an ever flowing river and how deeply we enter this river determines our experience of the water.

When not connected to this first body, there will not be a lot of abundance in any of your experiences. However as shown in the story about Guru Nanak and the farmer's field, when you are deeply connected to the first body you will live in the natural flow of abundance. The yogi realizes abundance, the unending flow of spirit, when all actions and projections are initiated from the energy of this first body, the soul body.

The first body is experienced when you live with humility. Humility is the spiritual quality that arises from mastering the first body. To experience humility you need to "bow" your head to your heart. Your mental process needs to be that you bow to the neutrality of your heart; only then will the ever-chattering, polarizing mind slow down so that the natural creativity of your soul can flow unimpeded.

When studying the lives of the mystics, we find that those who attained liberation from the constraints of their mind were from all walks of life. They exemplified that it doesn't matter what the external circumstances are, everyone has the same capacity to bow and to create that connection to their soul.

When you express the radiance of your soul with humility from bowing to the vastness of what is, then all the heavens are granted to you and the ultimate bliss of the universe is yours. You cannot buy this consciousness and no one outside of you can grant it. It is a state of being which you must claim, you must experience, "I am a beautiful spiritual being, I am, I am." This is the highest form of humble self-esteem.

It takes quite a bit of meditation to shift the energetic patterning from the old concepts and beliefs that we adapt from our culture and generational learning. One great concept to explore is this - your soul is actually a creative force. By observing your physical body and your life, you can tell whether you are really accessing the connection to your soul body. Only you can evaluate this. Only you can sit down and ask yourself how creative you are. Your creativity in how you flex with your life is the expression of the relationship to your soul.

I evaluate my first body periodically during the day by asking: "How creative am I? On a scale of 1 to 10, I am a 7." In such a case, I will do a yoga set or meditation to stimulate creativity, which comes from a connection to my soul. Eventually I will reach a point where I am so creative that I could write poetry. I could solve any problem - the solution just comes. We have observed that there are technologies to stimulate the soul body, for example you can do a yoga practice, or read JapJi Sahib, and be more creative.

So how do you evaluate your first body? One immediate way is to evaluate your physical body. Remember, the physical body just reflects the flow of your spirit. One very practical way to evaluate if you are in the flow is to observe if you get constipated. If so, it is a symptom that you have stopped the flow of spiritual energy in your body and your creative energy is stuck somewhere in your mind's process. At this point your mind is not reflecting the light of your soul, instead your mind is reflecting its unresolved karmic patterns. To keep the creative energy and bowels moving, you can take psyllium seed husks, flax seeds or chlorophyll.

When your soul body is working well then you will have excellent elimination. This eliminating force is called apana and is related to the creative energy, your kundalini. When your first body works you feel very creative about life. Once you are able to tune into your soul, the creative flow manifests as pure and blissful, because you know that you are one with Spirit and you experience the place of Spirit within yourself.

The first body aligns with the first chakra, the place where the kundalini ascends. All your creative force, your bija, is contained in the first chakra. It contains the basic nuclear energy of the human being - the power of the soul. There are lots of therapies and techniques to get the energy of the first chakra moving.

Reciting Japji Sahib, Asa Di Var, or the Mul Mantra stimulates your creative force and develops the connection to your soul body. It will unblock the energy of your soul so that you can experience your life as a Powerful, wonderful, creative flow.

What is it like to have creativity on command, to live in the space of unlimited creative force of the first body? Once you allow your mind to bow to your sacred heart, you will live in your ultimate spiritual expression. You will not need anything - money, love, power, security - because you have the ultimate relationship with your own soul and all your creativity flows.

"What are you doing? Your God is your spoken word. Shabad Guru. You are the disciple of the Shabad Guru. Nanak was the disciple of the Shabad Guru. You are the disciple of the Shabad Guru. Why should there be any difference between you and Nanak? We have the same teacher, the same thought, the same measurement, the same understanding. We look alike. We can talk alike. We can be alike"

- Yogi Bhajan 1992

"We don't worship Guru Nanak, we meditate on Guru Nanak"

-Yogi Bhajan 1994

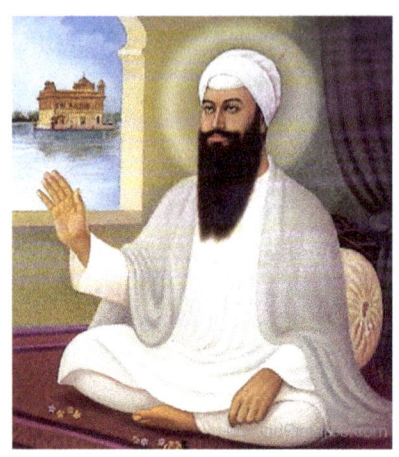

2
Second Body
Archetype: Guru Angad
Negative Mind
Containment, Obedience, Connected, Strategic

Guru Angad was born as Lehna in 1504. He was known for his obedience and devotion. Once, he was traveling on a pilgrimage to a Hindu shrine. While on his way, he learned that a holy man named Guru Nanak was working in a field along the way. He wanted to pay his respects, so he left the road and went into the field. As Lehna approached him, Guru Nanak called to him and requested that he help him by picking a big bundle of wet, muddy hay and carry it to a nearby house. Without hesitation, Lehna picked up the bundle, getting mud and straw all over his clothing.

Some of Guru Nanak's companions reproached him, saying, "You shouldn't have made him do that. He has ruined his robes." But Guru Nanak replied, "When you look at his clothes, you see mud, but I see something else. He hasn't carried a dirty burden. Rather, because of his obedience and devotion, he has washed his karmas. His name means ' he who is owed.' Now he has claimed what was meant to be his, this blessing." When Guru Nanak's companions looked again at Lehna, they saw no mud on him. Instead, his robe was splattered with saffron, the sign of blessings bestowed. In 1539, when Guru Nanak passed on the

Guruship to Guru Angad, he again splashed his robes with saffron. Guru Angad taught discipline, endurance, and steadfastness. By his example, he showed the dignity of honest labor and the importance of serving others before you take for yourself. He extended free kitchens and looked after the cooking and serving arrangements himself. He also developed the Gurumukhi script, which he used to record Guru Nanak's hymns as well as his own compositions. Guru Angad served until his death at age 48, in 1552.

Guru Angad is the archetype for the second body. This is the negative/protective facet of the mind, the first and fastest aspect of the three mental bodies. It gives the power of containment, form and discernment, which allows you to take the powerful creative force of the first body and express it in the form of enduring creations.

The creative force expressed by the soul body will be experienced as creative energy as it moves into the second body. Any activity in life is an external release of the creative energy from the first body. The second body is where your soul's energy starts to take form.

The second body corresponds to the second chakra, which is located in the reproductive organs and is ruled by the element of water. The water element helps things grow out of the earth of the first center. The element of water stimulates the longing to belong of the second center.

There are lots of ways to express the energy of the second body in relationship to someone else. You can play tennis, take a walk or create something together. The real question is this: how free flowing or how blocked is the energy circuit between the two of you? If you are in tune with your own soul and your creative energy is flowing, you can have that connection on a very high-level, soul to soul. It can be the subtlest interchange of energies - a look, a glance, a touch, or even the thought of each other during the day.

When you are tuned into your second body, you also develop an ability to connect with people at the level that they can hear you. It becomes your second nature to know how to create a connection with another person by using the subtleties of posture, gestures, tone of voice and facial expression. You know what kind of vocabulary to use, what you can talk about and what to avoid talking about.

A weak second body can make you awkward in your attempts to connect with people. You lack the flexibility needed to feel and approach their boundaries with grace. With a strong second center you can be highly creative about your connections.

The key to a healthy relationship with your second body is to develop the capacity to "listen". The most important and misused aspect of the mental bodies is this negative mind. Many get stuck in this protective process of the mind and are unable to move into the third body, the positive mind. All you see when you are stuck in the negative/protective aspect of the mind is insurmountable problems, conspiracy theories, and contraction.

The process of the 3 aspects of the mind starts here in the negative mind. We need to take time to pause and listen to the input of the negative mind, and then move the energy into the positive mind and then integrate the input from both the negative and the positive mind with the neutral mind.

This is true yoga, when you learn how to move thoughts, the impulses of your soul, THROUGH these three aspects of the mind.

Patanjali Rishi, who codified the yogic teachings, states the importance of this process in the second and third sutras:

Yogash chitta vritti nirodhah. Tada drashtuh svarupe avasthanam

'Yoga is experienced in that mind which has ceased to identify itself with its vacillating waves of perception, when this happens, then the Seer is revealed, resting in its own essential nature, and one realizes the True Self'

Once a successful businessman told me that he had lost $50,000 in the past nine years. Each year employees stole from him, one after the other. When I asked him if he checked into the backgrounds of his employees, he said, "Oh no, I always just follow my intuition." I asked him to trust his negative mind and to always do a background check. He did, and the problem was solved.

When your second body works well, you always take time to "listen." You ask yourself, "Okay, how do I cover myself if things are not as they seem or what do I do if things don't work out the way I hope and plan? **A well-known story to illustrate this point.**

There was once a man who was on his way back home from market with his camel and, as he had a good day, he decided to stop at a temple along the road and offer his thanks to God. He left his camel outside and went in with his prayer mat and spent several hours offering thanks to God, praying and promising that he would help the poor, and be an upstanding pillar of his community.

When he emerged it was already dark and – his camel was gone! He immediately flew into a violent temper and shook his fist at the sky, yelling: "You traitor! How could you do this to me? I put all my trust in you and then you go and stab me in the back like this!" A passing Sufi dervish heard the man yelling and told the man. "Listen," he said, "Trust God but, you know, tie up your camel."

In business and financial situations, the negative mind can serve you as it lets you know what could go wrong. It can calculate the danger in signing a financial contract, buying a new car, undertaking any transaction that involves profit and loss. It is the protective part of your mind that you often try to shut up while it yells at you, "That is too expensive! This is not really what I wanted! Something is off here!" It is important to remember that this protective expression is always the first aspect of the mind to engage. Learn to listen to its input first, and then engage the positive mind and the neutral mind (the third and fourth bodies) to balance it out to make a wise and informed decision. It is essential to use the early warning system of the negative mind to help you develop contingency plans and strategies in business and life. It is also essential to not get stuck in this aspect of the mind. Which could result in analysis paralysis.

How can you elevate your own second body? Look at your physical and emotional health. A weak second body can lead to physical symptoms such as kidney infections, urinary bladder infections, menstrual problems, diseases of the reproductive organs. These disorders all relate to how you use your second body to contain and give form to the creative energy of your being.

A weak second body is also indicated when someone has the habit of engaging in premature action. When you have a strong second body, you have the foresight and patience to wait for the right moment and the right conditions. Another symptom of a weak second body is being overly influenced by other people's realities, opinions, and personalities. Someone who has a weak second body is like a chameleon. They follow the crowd, try to fit in and don't listen enough to their own inner voice.

There are many natural therapies that will help to unblock your second body. Cucumber juice and nettle tea balance the bladder and kidneys and in some cases have even helped people pass kidney stones. There are also specific kundalini yoga sets for the kidneys. Chinese herbs and acupuncture are effective therapies to balance the second body.

Meditation, and the recitation of Shabad Hazare will harmonize the functioning of the second body.

The second body naturally matures with age because as people age they tend to slow down, listen and think about their responses and actions. They don't have all of the heat in their bodies that made them naturally impulsive and impatient when they were young. Age helps you gain experience and an understanding of the necessities of life, which gives you patience. When you master the second body you gain the quality of obeying your soul.

To most people, obedience has come to mean subjugating their will to someone else's will. The truest meaning of the word obedience is to listen to and obey your own soul. The second body helps you calculate the danger of listening to your ego instead of your soul, and this leads to obedience of the highest kind.

Once you have mastered your second body, you begin to enjoy ease in life. You have gained the true relaxation that comes from an obedient relationship to your soul. You develop trust in yourself to use your protective, negative mind to cover every situation gracefully. And you have the patience, timing and wisdom that allow you to savor every moment and every experience as a gift from the Infinite.

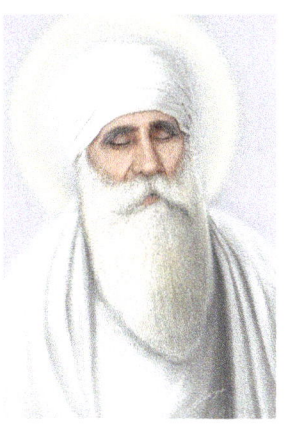

3
Third Body
Archetype: Guru Amar Das
Positive/Projective Mind
Positivity, Equality, Thy Will is My Will

Guru Amar Das was born in 1479. He was crowned as the Guru very late in life, at the age of 73. He earned this great blessing through his devotion to Guru Angad. Every day, rain or shine, Amar Das brought water to Guru Angad for his bath. He had to walk five miles to the river and then five miles back again, carrying a heavy bucket of water on his head. One day, when he was already an old man, he was returning from the river during a rainstorm with his load of water. He slipped and fell in the mud outside the home of a weaver. The weaver heard the noise of his fall and asked his wife, "Has someone had an accident?" She replied sarcastically, "who else but Amar Das? He is like a mule, carrying water every day. He acts like a slave!"

When Amar Das returned to the Gurus Home, Guru Angad asked him, "Are you all right? Did something happen to you?" Amar Das replied, " Guru, you know everything. I am fine. Everything is all right." Then the Guru said, "People have said you are a slave and have no honor, but you will be the honor of every human being and bestow honor on all. People have said that you have no home, but you will provide homes for everyone. People have said that you have no one who loves you, but you will become the beloved of all who connect with you." Guru Angad blessed Amar Das and said, "Because of your selfless service and devotion, you will be the next Guru."

Guru Amar Das collected the hymns of Guru Nanak and Guru Angad, as well as writing many poetic songs of divine love and devotion himself. Guru Amar Das instituted lungar programs, so that all people, no matter what caste they were from, could share food. To this day at the Golden Temple all who come for food sit on the floor together and are served the same food.

During his leadership he further established Sikh Dharma organizationally, and worked to promote the cause of women's dignity and equality. He served until his death at the age of 95, in 1574.

The life of Guru Amar Das exemplifies the third body. It is your projective, positive mind. It allows you to direct the light of your soul beyond the negative and observe the positive essence of all situations and all beings. Your third body corresponds to your navel center. It is the center of your power, your digestive fire and will. Once this power center is open, you experience your connection to the One constant source. This experience of equality allows you to see that everyone has the same capacity within themselves to be great, to be exalted, to discover and express their own infinity. The capacity to see all beings as Sat Nam, Pure Spirit, is the expression of a strong third body. You see all as truly equal in the opportunity to express their potential.

With a strong third body, you have the capacity to see all people as equal. You can un-see their negativity and get past their exterior projections. With a strong third body you easily see another's positive essence and recognize their soul. This ability frees you up to use your own power to serve. When you are in the flow of infinite power, you become personally powerful, and you live to share your strength with others.

When your third body is fully developed you emanate a sense of power in a humble way. Your body is fit, your weight is balanced, your skin is radiant, your mind is powerful and your communication is strong and direct. Everybody in the family can be complaining about someone, and you find something genuinely positive to say about that person. You always find some positive quality to attribute to any person. You take any situation and find something positive in it. You can see the humor in the play of life.

The third center is the maleness of your being, whether you are male or female. It is the power center, the fire in the belly. Sometimes people are afraid of their own power, afraid of the responsibility it brings, or they are afraid that they will abuse power. Maybe someone abused them and they try to block their own power center out of unresolved fear. People with a blocked third center are not using their own 'heat'. They typically are overweight, sluggish, depressed, passive, disorganized, and lack in will. If you do not have a strong third center your negative mind can take over your mental processing to the point that it paralyzes you with its negativity and you just want to give up. If you don't engage the positive mind appropriately it will only be able to magnify the problems, which the second body identifies. The positive mind needs to be engaged to identify and magnify new possibilities and opportunities. Without the conscious application of your will, the positive mind can actually cause you to lose more of your will and power.

The journey to create a strong, balanced third body is intense because to open up and receive the hope and positivity which a strong third body gives, you have to burst through all of the depression and negative thoughts that you energetically hold in your self-experience. The third center is also very challenging as it invokes your true power once you have integrated the negative experiences in your relationship to power.

People with the opposite imbalance in their power center will be very thin. They are so willful and inflexible that it eats them up. These people have so much fire that they get too hot. We all know people like that - they have a perfect spiritual discipline for a while, but they are doing it from a place that is so dogmatic and tense that it eventually burns them out. The most sustainable balance in the third body comes when you have the fire from the third center kept in balance with enough water from the second center.

Some physical symptoms that can occur with an unbalanced third body are liver and gallbladder dysfunctions, ankle and foot pain, cramps, weak eyes, headaches, allergies, and low back pain. Typical emotional states of an imbalanced third center are anger, intolerance, and depression. Yogic therapies to balance the third center are yoga sets for the liver, stretch pose, and meditations that activate the navel center.

A powerful way to strengthen the positive mind is to read Guru Amar Das bani, to chant Anand Sahib and to recite the Ardas Bhayee mantra. You can also practice affirmations to open up to positive changes in your life. Affirmations are just simple, direct statements affirming your intended reality. Do not make an affirmation reflect how things are already, instead describe the ultimate state of *being* that you want to reach.

When you construct an affirmation, say exactly what you want rather than what you don't want. You will get better at doing this as your positive mind gets stronger. People who are not used to applying their positive minds in this way will actually end up affirming what they don't want. For instance, if you are playing golf you might say to yourself, "Don't hit the ball in the water." Your mind is more likely to respond to the concrete realities of "ball" and "water" than to the abstraction of "don't". And if you think it enough, your obedient mind may send your ball right into the water!

Instead of saying, "don't" or "not" or "won't", be directly descriptive of what it is you DO want. "I am going to hit my ball right onto the green of the fifth hole and it will roll right into the cup."

There is a great story about Guru Gobind Singh in an archery competition. The target was a flower and the bull's-eye was the center of that small flower. The Guru won the contest. Someone asked him where he had aimed and he said: "I aimed for the center of that flower". It sounds obvious, but it's amazing how often we don't do that.

Sometimes people have an immediate negative reaction to affirmations. As soon as they hear themselves say the affirmation, they think, "That is ridiculous: I am not happy; I am not prosperous; I am not successful." It makes them feel stupid to say something that goes so against their programming. Yet that is the whole point. If you have a negative emotional response to an affirmation like, "I am happy," you know that you have triggered a karmic button and discovered one of your negative programs. Then you can use an affirmation to replace the old program with something more productive. Think of it like programming a computer. If your computer does something that is not effective, you know that you have discovered a glitch in the program it is using. You then have to get in there and replace the old message with the new one. Your infinite mind works like that as well.

One easy way to get past your initial negative response to affirmations is to make a recording in your own voice. Play the recording continuously in the evening while you sleep, keep the volume low so you can barely hear it. The subconscious mind will accept the affirmation without the fight the conscious mind might put up. Listening to recordings in your own voice while you sleep is a way to bypass the conscious mind and deeply imprint the subconscious mind. You know that the affirmations have begun to empower the third body when you start to exhibit new behaviors. You may find that initially when you start to sleep to these affirmations, your sleep will be a little restless. You will get used to this "reprogramming" fairly quickly. Mystics know that our own voice is actually our favorite sound.

For instance, for me it was a leap to say to myself, "I am a yogi." It brought up all my self-esteem and success issues. So I made a recording in my own voice saying the positive affirmation, "I am a yogi," and I listened to it every night for a while. As the affirmation sank into my unconscious, I went through big changes. I began to feel like a yogi; I began to act like a yogi; I began to speak to people to share universal knowledge. When I started using affirmations to strengthen that identity, it sped up the process of empowering the third body and I consciously directed all the creative fire from this body to be a yogi.

You might find that when you are ready to expand your emotional beliefs into a bigger space you will experience a lot of conflict. That is because you are taking an established pattern in your subconscious mind that has been a survival tool for you and saying, "that is limited and I choose to expand." Changing karmic beliefs is like a baby bird jumping out of the nest for the first time. It does not even know it has wings, and only when falling does it find its wings. We won't use our greatest talents until we can let go of what was and grow the wings we need to serve the new reality.

Your karmic/emotional beliefs are contained in organic matter - the brain - and you cannot delete an energetic pattern without uploading a new pattern to take its place. That is where yoga and meditation come in. With bani and mantra (sacred sounds), pranayam (yogic breathing) and asanas (postures), you can create enough psychic heat (*tapasia*) to shift karmic patterns that don't resonate with your soul.

When you affirm your new identity for forty days, it will start to affect your consciousness. Practice it for ninety days and your new identity will start to shine through more than your old one. Practice it for one hundred and twenty days and your new identity will be fully established and the old pattern will be replaced. To permanently experience your own positivity and balanced power, direct the fire of the third body by reading bani and affirmations, practicing a yoga set and meditation every day for four months.

"Put on Ardas Bhayee mantra. This is the most powerful combination and permutation of sound current of Shabad. It penetrates through all that there is. Ardas Bhayee, Amar Das Guru, Amar Das Guru Ardas Bhayee. Ram Das Guru Ram Das Guru Ram Das Guru, Sachee Sahee. Sing with it. Instead of complaining - chant. Guru Amar Das is bhandari. Bhandari is the one who maintains you, sustains you. He is bhandari and Guru Ram Das is the Lord of Miracles. So, when we say this – these are the very exact words – Ardas Bhayee, a prayer has happened. You are not praying; this very intention to pray is the micro-consciousness. Your consciousness is already confirming it"

-Yogi Bhajan 1999

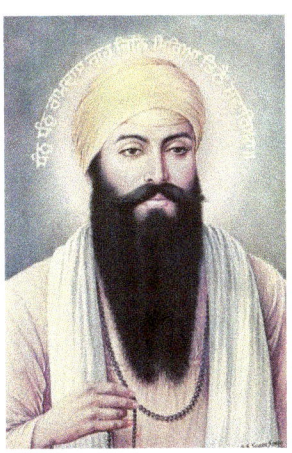

4
Fourth Body
Archetype: Guru Ram Das
Neutral Mind
Compassion, Integration, Service

Guru Ram Das was born in 1534 as Jetha. He was orphaned early in life, and spent his days selling wheat berries outside the house of Guru Amar Das. After selling his wares all day long, he would stay near the Guru late into the night, cooking langar and washing the feet of those who came to receive the Guru's blessings. Guru Amar Das and his wife grew to love Jetha deeply. When it was time for their daughter, Bibi Bani, to get married Guru Amar Das asked his wife, "Who should our daughter marry?" and she replied "Only someone who is as selfless and loving as Jetha." "Yes" replied Guru Amar Das, "there is no one else as selfless and loving as he." Before his death, Guru Amar Das bestowed the Guruship on his son-in-law, and named him Guru Ram Das.

Guru Ram Das established the Sikh center, Ram Das Pur, which is now known as Amritsar. Seekers would travel to that city to be with the Guru and receive his blessing. Guru Ram Das was the living embodiment of humility and service. At night, he would go to the houses where the pilgrims were resting and would wash and massage their feet and serve them food. One day some people came to a rest house in Ram Das Pur. A very humble man served them food, made their beds up for them, and massaged their feet. In the morning the people went to the Guru's court to receive his blessing. As they peered through the crowd to watch a glimpse of him, they were shocked to see that the man sitting on the Guru's throne was the same man who had served them the night before. They exclaimed, "We came to serve you but you have served us with your own hands!"

Guru Ram Das was a raj yogi – he integrated nobility, royalty and spiritual discipline with the humbleness of a family person's life. He taught his students to wake before the sun rises to chant bani and sit in meditation. His life demonstrated how to live in this world, but not be off it.

Guru Ram Das wrote beautiful poetry and songs of devotion, including the Lavan, which is sung during the Sikh wedding ceremony. He began construction of the Golden Temple and supervised the work himself. Guru Ram Das left his body in 1581, at the age of 47.

The life of Guru Ram Das demonstrates the mastery of the fourth Body. The fourth body is the neutral mind. It corresponds to the heart chakra and directs the entire capacity of the human being. The neutral mind is the mind of a sant and yogi - it looks at the input of the negative mind for what could go wrong and then gets input from the positive mind for what could go right and then it integrates the information in accordance with the soul's highest expression. It articulates the ultimate win-win mentality.

The fourth body integrates all of the other bodies; it evaluates them for their input within nine seconds, and only then gives you an answer. Your neutral mind allows you to see the big picture so that you can respond and not react. This integration allows you to rise above personal agendas so that you can easily access your soul. The fourth body is a very exalted space - from this vantage point you can look with compassion on the whole play of life.

The neutral mind gives you the ability to see through *Maya*, the illusion of this worldly manifestation. With a strong neutral mind you know that when you die you will not be taking your money or your job or your family with you - you will be alone, to face your own supreme Self. The connection to your higher self is very integrated when the neutral mind is strong.

When you live and operate from the awareness of the neutral mind, it gives you a mind which observes possibilities versus polarities. You still live life with its ups and downs. You still have feelings, both positive and negative. But as you learn to rely more and more on your fourth body, your emotions and commotions get integrated and transformed into devotion. You now elevate your emotional energy into compassion and kindness. This compassion is for the soul's journey, not to be confused with empathy for the ego's drama. Compassion expressed through a balanced fourth body is very direct and clear. It does not cater to ego.

With a balanced fourth body you realize that everything is perfect just as it is, you appreciate the present, and you know that every moment of life holds a valuable lesson. You let the events of life unfold and play themselves out, you trust the process.

One way to activate the heart center is to chant Guru Ram Das Bani. This sacred sound activates the heart chakra, and when the neutral mind's frequency dominates, it puts you in a harmonic state with your soul. The expression of the integrated neutral mind allows you to manifest life as a pure being.

When you master your fourth body you do not have regrets; you do not look at things in terms of the polarities of right and wrong. You see how to integrate your current experiences and know that every event in your life is for your benefit, each event makes you wiser. Life is happening for you, not to you.

Love of *seva*, selfless service, is another quality of the fourth body. We all do service at some point in our lives and often we are doing it from a state where our egos have an agenda. Some examples: "I did such a good job; everyone will be impressed." "I am a good person now that I have worked so hard." "I am needed - if I do not do it, it will not get done." "I did it perfectly." "I wish I could be doing something else." "Why is so-and-so not here to help me?" "Maybe I will just do it halfway and get out of here sooner." "What does it matter if I am doing this, it will just get wrecked again in an hour." "This doesn't really need to be done, who said it did?"

There is nothing wrong with having any of these thoughts or feelings. That is what the mind does; it judges constantly and you need your mind in order to live in a human body. Judging yourself or trying to use your will to overcome these thoughts will not stop your mind from chattering away at you. Just relax about it, and as we say, "be the observer and pass the popcorn." Become aware of the thoughts and feelings that arise and demand your attention - just watch them and have compassion for your human ego. At the same time, become more and more aware of the part of you that just serves, the part that exists in the timeless space where service just is and you are in the flow of it. That is the real gift of *seva* - instead of being in the limited space of your ego, you dwell in the blissful, infinite space of the flow of the neutral mind through service.

The fourth body corresponds to the fourth chakra and is also called the "cup of prayer." It acts as the guiding force for the other nine bodies. The integrated ten-body process is to check in with all ten bodies and then to act through the fourth body.

I have learned to trust my fourth body to guide me, so that I listen to my soul even when I may not know the eventual outcome. I took on the seva of building a Gurdwara in Espanola, New Mexico, because I felt it would have an integrative effect on the community. I was willing to sacrifice and go through mental and financial hardship. It took me a year to recover from all of that, probably because my ego was so invested. But that is not necessarily a negative thing. I used my ego to serve a higher purpose. While in this body, you can never be devoid of ego, but you can put your ego to the service of a higher function. The key is whether you can recognize that Spirit is acting through you and that some things are destined to flow through you.

Someone with an imbalanced fourth body might have uneven facial features or other asymmetries in the body because the two hemispheres of the brain are not balanced. Dyslexia and other learning disorders arise when the left and right brain don't communicate. There can also be diaphragm tightness, breathing problems, irregular heartbeat, or hiatal hernia.

When the fourth body is off-balance, you have a hard time integrating experiences and finding meaning. "Why did that happen to me? I did not deserve that." You do not recognize that everything in life has a greater purpose. Fear, anger, sadness, and victimization are the symptoms of the inability to integrate events in a yogic way. Western culture tends to see life in terms of right and wrong. It is difficult to integrate events if they are believed to be either black or white. It is hard to observe everything as a lesson if everything has to be either right or wrong. Many Westerners do not naturally have a strong neutral mind and they need to consciously develop it.

One day I was treating a woman in my office and my intuition told me, "Just listen to her and don't speak yet." As a healer, I have learned to use my neutral mind to hear not just the words the person is saying, but also what the psyche is saying. This woman was saying, "My back hurts here, and when I twist this way it hurts here," but as she was saying these words, all I could hear was, "She has been abused and she doesn't remember it, but don't tell her yet. She will not be able to handle it right now." So I wrote down the details of her complaints and her medical history. I knew in my heart that her real pain was coming from that abuse. My intuition helped me by telling me to listen carefully with my neutral mind. And my neutral mind told me what to do with that knowledge. Receiving information with your intuition is the first step, then it has to be balanced by the neutral mind so that you know what to do with it.

I treated this woman twice a week for three months and then once a week for the next three months. Six months after I first met her, she walked into my office and said: "Dr. Khalsa, you know, I feel 95% better, but there is this one pain…" At this point my neutral mind told me "Now you can tell her she was abused." I could have let fear come in at that point, but I trusted my fourth body, so I said, "Well, you have that pain because when you were a very young girl you were abused." The woman cried for three hours and then a bump came up right on the acupuncture point that stores old trauma. She said to me, "I never told anyone." One week before she came to see me, the uncle who had abused her was dying. On his deathbed he looked up at her and asked,

"Have you forgiven me?" This had triggered all of her old memories about the event.

As a healer, what I needed in that situation was a strong neutral mind. I did not need to evaluate anything or to psychoanalyze her experience. I needed to listen to my neutral mind and obey its direction.

Once a friend of mine kept telling me all the negatives that had been going on in his life. I could have responded by helping him see the positives in order to give him hope; instead my neutral mind told me, confront him! Help him break this continuous negative cycle. Because of my relationship with my fourth body, I trusted that voice in me and I let the confrontation flow through me. I trusted that it would be in my friend's best interest, and it was.

When you access your neutral mind (the fourth body) you can command it to override whatever keeps you from being creative. A strong fourth body gives you the ability to integrate the polarities of life. It allows you to go beyond either/or and get to both/and. It lets you see the apparent contradictions of life as paradox. The fourth body has no gender; it is that state of purity beyond the dualities of positive and negative. It also gives you the capacity to return from that infinite space of no duality and recognize the here and now.

There are some very powerful yogic therapies to strengthen the fourth body, so you can experience balance and neutrality. Kirtan Kriya or Sa Ta Na Ma meditation balances all five *tattvas*, or elements, and also the brain hemispheres. Cross-crawl exercises actually inspire the corpus callussum of the brain to make connecting fibers between the two hemispheres. There are also specific hemisphere-balancing meditations. You can meditate on yogic mandalas as the pattern in a mandala guides your brain into a neutral space. You can also read Guru Ram Das bani, and Tav Prasad Swayaia, and do seva.

The process of creating a neutral integrated expression from all of life's events is the yogi's journey. When you no longer participate in the reactivity of karma, by integrating the negative and positive charged emotions, then you can truly serve humanity. You are neutral not to be confused with neutered. A strong fourth center expresses as engaged and powerful, not accommodating or disconnected. You express the light of your soul with balanced power in a clear, and direct way. You do not need recognition; you do not need rewards. You do not need anything because you already have it all.

"Now, Guru Ram Das rules the heart center. Guru Ram Das is a very, very good guru. Funny in many ways. There is one problem you have to understand. Nank too lehenaa too hai, guru amar too vecharia. The three combinations in the fourth opens the heart center, that is the base. The Asan. From there onwards it rules. So basically he rules the 10 bodies."

-Yogi Bhajan 1985

Student: "What test must each of the 10 bodies pass through for the soul to achieve liberation?"

Yogi Bhajan: "Neutral mind. Meditative mind is the answer."

- Yogi Bhajan 1981

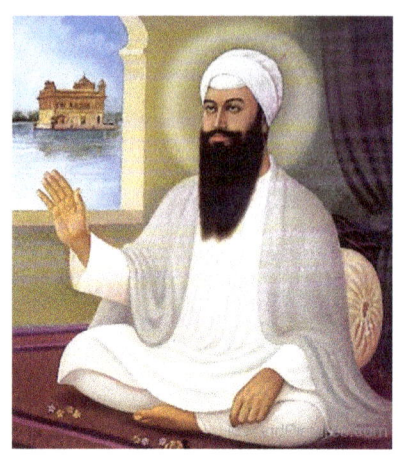

5
Fifth Body
Archetype: Guru Arjan
Physical Body
Balance, Sacrifice, Teacher

Guru Arjan Dev, born in 1563, was the youngest son of Guru Ram Das. Arjan Dev loved to serve his father. Once Guru Ram Das sent Arjan Dev to another town to attend the wedding of a friend and told him, "Stay there until I call for you to return." After a few months of being apart from his beloved Guru and father, Arjan Dev could no longer bear the separation. He wrote two letters full of longing and devotion to Guru Ram Das and sent them to him by messenger.

But when the letters reached the Guru's court they were intercepted by Arjan Dev's older brother, who envied his younger brother and wanted to become the next Guru. After awaiting a reply from his Guru and not receiving one, Arjan Dev wrote another letter of love and longing, requesting to come home. This one reached Guru Ram Das and he read it. When the Guru discovered that his youngest son had written two letters that had never reached him, he inquired throughout his household, "Who has taken these letters?" But everyone denied any involvement. Eventually, the two missing letters were found in the coat pocket that belonged to Arjan Dev's older brother. When confronted by the Guru, he claimed that he himself had written those beautiful letters of devotion. "Very well," said his father and Guru, "Write another one just like these two." But the older brother could not do it – he didn't have the devotion and longing to create such letters full of love. Guru Ram Das sent for Arjan Dev, asking him to return home. When he arrived, he was filled with bliss at the presence of his bellowed Guru, and wrote a fourth letter. In response to his son's devotion, Guru Ram Das crowned him as Guru Arjan Dev in 1581, when he was only 18 years old.

Guru Arjan Dev's commitment to harmony and justice enraged the oppressive Muslim king, who sentenced Guru Arjan Dev to sit on a burning, hot plate and be covered in hot sand. Guru Arjan Dev endured this torture without a word of complaint or a hint of pain. After two-and-a-half days, he asked if he could take a dip in the river. Thinking that the water would only increase his pain and suffering, the Muslim king agreed to let him do it. Guru Arjan Dev was carried to the water and put into it. He sank beneath the surface and never returned.

Guru Arjan Dev oversaw the completion of the Golden Temple. The temple is build half of marble and half of gold and is a physical representation of the balance, which Guru Arjan Dev demonstrated in his life.

His greatest contribution to the Sikh way of life was the compilation of the Adi Granth, later to become the Siri Guru Granth Sahib the living Sikh Guru. Arjan Dev affirmed the unified quality of all mystic experience as he included the writings of the Sikh Gurus as well as Hindu bhaktas, Muslim pirs, Sufi poets and other realized beings.

Reflect on these writings of Guru Arjan, the archetype for the fifth Body:

Sukhmani Sahib:
"The whole world of being is contained within the One, who appears as many in His manifold play. The Nectar-Name is the source of every conceivable joy. And it lives within the body."

"Ang Sang Wahe Guru", in every part of my physical presence, I experience bliss.

The ultimate expression of the fifth body is to realize this balance between the physical and the eternal and to experience this at every moment, with every breath.

Guru Arjan's martyrdom occurred in 1606 when he was 43 years old. Your fifth body is your physical body, the one that everyone sees, the one through which the other nine bodies can play out their parts. When you have a strong fifth center you are balanced in your life and you know the Balance of Life.

What does it mean to be balanced? If you work seven days a week, to create more balance you could choose to disconnect from your phone and Internet from 8pm until 8am every day. If your eating habits are out of harmony, and you want to create more balance, you could choose to fast for one day each week. A person who is balanced knows their capacity and takes alone time to regenerate. How yogis take this time daily is in the early morning hours, the amrit vela, with yoga and meditation.

To keep balance in a yoga practice, do both the asanas and the long deep relaxation. So many people do the asanas and then jump right into their busy lives again without taking the time to integrate the effects of the asanas and balance 'doing with being'. Also be mindful to balance the practices which support you personally, with practices to connect to group consciousness and practices that connects you to universal consciousness.

Here are some examples on how you could do this:

- **Personal:** Daily early morning yoga set and meditation.
- **Group:** Attending community yoga classes and doing seva.
- **Universal:** Offering a prayer at an altar for global transformation/healing.

To keep your life in balance you need to look at how you use your time and energy. How much is for you? How much is for your community commitments? How much is for your family? How much is for your business? There is a balance you need to maintain so that you get the right amount of yoga, meditation, exercise, water and food, sleep, intimacy, work, relaxation, contemplation, social time, privacy - all of the elements of a healthy life. Make sure that everything is dealt with in a balanced way; even with the seemingly mundane things like rushing when going to the bathroom or overeating. This or any lack of balance always impacts the overall strength of your fifth body.

When your fifth body is working for you, you have the capacity to sacrifice. In modern culture, we have come to think of sacrifice as drudgery, as giving up something we really want. In recent times, our culture has encouraged people to always satisfy themselves instantly and never to do without. A strong fifth center gives you the awareness that something you want today could jeopardize something more important in the future. A strong fifth center gives the ability to see enough of the balance of life so that you can give up something in order to keep things in a higher state of balance. Self-sacrifice does not mean taking care of everyone else and not yourself. It means sacrificing your selfish desires so that your higher self can serve a greater cause.

When you have a strong fifth center you can sacrifice your own convenience for the higher benefit of others when that is what is needed. If your friend calls you at night during your favorite TV program, and says, "I have just had a horrible experience. Please come over, I have to talk to you," you go right away without a second thought. Those with a weak fifth body would say, "I don't have time for that stuff. I am too busy. I work eighty hours a week, I need to relax now." A person like that probably doesn't want to be selfish. But if he works eighty hours a week, his life is so out of balance that he can't see beyond his own nose. Balancing your life makes room for you to be able to sacrifice with grace when needed.

When your fifth body, your throat chakra, is strong you will speak eloquently. You have a great range of flexibility in your capacity to communicate, and you have the natural ability to know when to speak and went to be silent. Again, a sense of balance is the key. When your fifth center is powerful, you will naturally share what you know through teaching.

Teaching involves sacrifice. To be a teacher requires that you hold the space to reflect the highest potential of the person you are with and not drop into any "pity-party" or political conversations. As Kundalini Yoga teachers we take a vow before we teach: "I am not a woman, I am not a man, I am not a person, I am not myself, I am a teacher." This mantra creates a pure connection to the fifth body, the body of the teacher. Then as a teacher you use the power of your words to inspire, which sometimes means you have to say that which is not popular or warm and fuzzy. Once you commit to hold this sacred space of a teacher, you will be able to do so with everyone all the time.

When you have a strong fifth center you are balanced – not too thin, not overweight, right in the balanced middle. You have balanced facial features and a good sense of balance in your physical body.

How would I know if someone's fifth body was weak? I would ask her: "Do you teach anything? Do you enjoy showing people how to do things?" Everyone has something they can teach. Most of the time, when someone comes to me needing healing, something is out of balance in his or her life. I am always looking for what that is. She has disrupted her harmony somewhere and that harmony needs to be restored. She needs to balance all the parts of her life. For example, if you put in sixty hours a week for a while, then you better take your partner on vacation the next month or you are going to experience the drama of imbalance.

The fifth center is located at the thyroid gland. When your fifth body is out of balance, your thyroid could start malfunctioning. You can get metabolism problems, growth problems, or neck problems. Thyroid imbalance can also cause disturbances in the heart and small intestine.

When your fifth chakra, the throat chakra, is blocked, you may have problems with your speech. Connect the thumb of your right hand to the pinkie finger of your right hand and then make the same mudra with your left hand (Buddhi Mudra). Chant the mantra: *"RA RA RA RA, MA MA MA MA, RAMA RAMA RAMA RAMA SA TA NA MA."* I have seen this meditation cure people of stuttering. It harmonizes the two hemispheres of the brain by balancing the incoming communication of the left hand and the outgoing communication of the right-hand. Any chanting of banis or mantras will harmonize this body, especially Sukhmani Sahib, and the Ad Guray Nameh mantra,

To keep the fifth body strong and balanced, exercise a minimum of half an hour three times a week. That is the minimum; an hour per day would be optimal. You also need at least half an hour of yoga each day and aerobic exercise three times a week. You have to put that kind of energy out to keep your fifth body strong so that, when the opportunity comes, the balance between your will and your feelings will allow you to make the required sacrifice. The word sacrifice comes from the Latin word *sacrificium*, which means, "to make sacred." That is the true gift of the strong fifth body - you live your life in such balance and harmony that you come to the realization that every part of life is sacred.

"That is why Guru Nanak became Guru by the Shabad Guru. That is why we worship Shabad Guru today. So each individual is sovereign. Each individual is the creator's creation. Each individual is atma. Each individual has to recognize pavan guru. Pavan guru means prana's guru. And that is Shabad. When you repeat the shabad, when you speak, it affects, it projects and it relates. If your words are that of God, they are infinite. If your words are that of earth, the are limited."

- Yogi Bhajan 1994

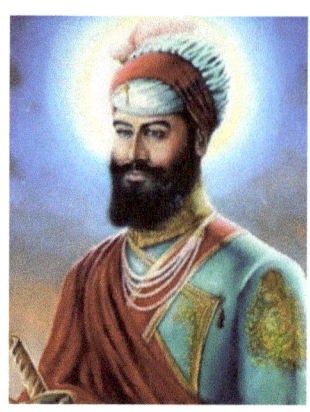

6
The Sixth Body
Archetype: Guru Hargobind
The Arc Line
Protection, Projection, Intuition

Guru Hargobind, born in 1595, was Guru Arjan Dev's son. He became Guru when he was 11 years old. During the succession ceremony he said, "I will wear two swords. One symbolizes spirituality (Piri); the other symbolizes strength and worldly leadership (Miri). I shall live royally and so shall my Sikhs. We stand firm against injustice and are prepared to defend honor." Guru Hargobind furthered the development of the Sikh sovereign community by establishing the Akal Takhat next to the Golden Temple to create that balance of Miri represented by the Akal Takhat and Piri represented by the Golden Temple. Guru Hargobind had a powerful spiritual practice and also raised an army to protect sovereignty and defend justice.

The Muslim emperor, Jahangir, was concerned about Guru Hargobind's power. He had the Guru arrested and put into a cell in Gwalior Fort along with 52 princes who had also been unjustly detained. One day a Muslim saint came to the palace for an audience with the emperor. He told him, "You have made a grave error by imprisoning such a great saint. This injustice will destroy your kingdom." The emperor became alarmed and ordered that Guru Hargobind be released. But the Guru refused to leave unless the other 52 prisoners were released as well.

Thinking to appease him, the emperor agreed that anyone who could hold on to the Guru's robes as he walked out of the prison would be allowed to accompany him to freedom. In response, Guru Hargobind asked his Sikhs to make a special robe for him, a robe with 52 separate panels. Despite the fact that he was free to leave, he waited at the prison until the robe was completed. When that day arrived, he walked out of Gwalior Fort accompanied by his 52 fellow prisoners, each one holding on to a panel of his robe. Guru Hargobind left his body in 1644, at the age of 49.

The sixth body is the arc line, which connects earlobe to earlobe over the forehead. Just as the life of Guru Hargobind demonstrated the balance between the physical and the cosmic realms, between Miri and Piri, the 6th body integrates the inflow of cosmic experience from the subtle bodies with the physical experience of the first five bodies.

The sixth body corresponds to the pituitary gland, the master gland of the endocrine system. The sixth body controls the nervous system and the glands. The sixth chakra rules the pericardium meridian, which protects the heart center and glands, and the triple heater meridian, which also relates to the glands. A balanced sixth body manifests as having powerful intuition, which protects the heart center and allows you to live with an open heart. It makes your glandular system strong, which makes your nervous system strong, which lets you deal with the stresses of life without having to shut down your heart.

When the intuitive knowing from the sixth body, the arc line, protects your heart center, you are self-assured, open and loving. You are also self-reliant; if there is some danger you take charge of the situation and handle it. Someone whose sixth center is functioning well makes statements like: "I am always in the right place at the right time, things flow so easily for me, everything I do just works out. " That person is crisp, articulate, and focused. When you talk to them, they are very present.

There are two aspects to the sixth body: protection and projection. The intuition of the sixth center protects by telling you what is coming at you. When driving down the street, you will get the urge to turn at the next street. That night while watching the news you find out that by turning at that street you avoided sitting in traffic for an hour.

Sometimes you get a feeling about a person or a situation and later realize that the feeling kept you from getting involved in something destructive. Your intuition protects you when you have a clear relationship to the sixth body.

When you consciously choose to listen to your intuition, it gives you inner confirmation of your psychic sense. When you trust your intuition 100%, then you listen to your soul. Whether it is true or not true to other people does not matter to you, because that is not what you trust. You trust the relationship with your own inner Self.

A strong sixth body gives intuitive knowing in relationship with your partner. This is important because she/he has such direct access to your heart. You will typically get into an argument with your partner when you have not bothered to tune into the space she/he is in that day. You start a conversation without being alert, aware, or sensitive. Once you can use your intuition, you won't have to shut down your heart as a way to defend yourself. A strong sixth body gives the capacity to hold the projection of the long term intention for being in relationship vs. wanting to be right in the fight.

The arc line also gives the power of projection; the capacity to manifest those things you want in your life. It focuses your projection and aligns it with your sense of sacredness. When you know that you are at one with Spirit, whatever you project manifests. It is only when you separate yourself and think that Spirit's will and your will are different that you cannot manifest. With a clear sixth body there is no separation between your will and Spirit's will. With a strong sixth body you are a total flow of Spirit.

Actually, both protection and projection are happening simultaneously. The arc line is the external projective part of the third eye. Internally at the third eye, you audit all the information and put it into your total psyche and hear the answer. Externally, you project your intention out so clearly that the universe responds.

The sixth center is also referred to as a "person at prayer," someone whose inner life is in the constant flow of the intuitive Self. Your being is a living prayer, a manifestation, not a doing or an asking for something.

A 'person at prayer' lives the experience that their inner vibratory frequency is what manifests their outer reality.

An imbalance in the sixth body leads to glandular imbalances. Any kind of glandular imbalance leads to behavior dysfunction. Your mind will jump around - monkey mind - and it will be impossible to focus. You find it difficult to keep your personality in an even flow, to have your behavior be consistent and constant. In extreme forms, this can manifest as manic depression.

'So Darshan Chakra Kriya' meditation is a great way to balance and strengthen the sixth center. The depth of your meditative capacity is based on the strength of your navel. That is why 'So Darshan Chakra Kriya' is powerful; it connects the third center and the sixth center so that the power of your projection can come through. 'So Darshan Chakra Kriya' helps you take all of the energy you have developed in your higher centers and brings it down into your body to manifest onto the earth.

With a strong sixth body all you have to do to realize what you intend is to really focus on it. When you develop your sixth center you have that kind of focus. You set an intention and it manifests. You just intend for something and it happens. You get constant confirmation that you are one with the universe; you are the living proof of this over and over and over. You honor and respect each word and thought as a prayer, an energetic projection that will live forever in the akashic records.

"When the Guru sits in the heart, it doesn't matter what is written in the destiny. If the word of the Guru sits in your heart, whatever is written on your forehead shall be re-written automatically, you have to do nothing about it"

- Yogi Bhajan 1983

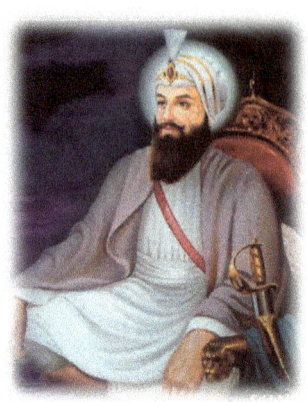

7
The Seventh Body
Archetype: Guru Har Rai
The Aura
Security, Love, Kindness

Guru Har Rai was born in 1630 and became Guru at the age of 14, in 1644. He was in charge during a peaceful era in India, and he devoted his energy to travel, teach, and form the Sikhs into a close-knit community. He dedicated himself to meditate and was known for his personal discipline.

During his travels, Guru Har Rai stopped late one night at the house of a poor family. He said to the woman of the house, "Dear sister, I am so hungry. Please bring me the bread you have made for me." The woman was overjoyed to serve him the coarse bread she had prepared, and he ate it eagerly while still sitting on his horse. After thanking and blessing the woman, the Guru continued on his journey.

His disciples were amazed at his departure from his usual discipline and they questioned him. He laughed and replied, "What caused me to beg for the bread was not the hunger of my stomach, but my hunger for the song of love with which the bread was made. Seldom do I get such bread. I am pulled by the strings of love. God is love."

It is said that when Guru Har Rai realized that his youngest son was the next embodiment of Guru Nanak, he bowed down to him and left his body. He died in 1661, at the age of 31.

The seventh body is your aura, the electromagnetic field around your body. It emanates from the tenth gate, the crown chakra which is open at the time of birth and then closes as we age. The degree of openness of this chakra determines the strength of the seventh body, the aura. It gives you the capacity to dwell in the experience of love which Guru Har Rai embodied, and to feel the security of your spiritual identity. A strong aura lets you feel safe and secure. It is your energetic envelope, like a constant hug by the divine mother energy of the universe. This sense of security allows you connect to your heart and to be loving and kind with yourself and others.

Your aura is created by the flow of energy that goes through the meridian system of the body. Prana comes in through the tenth gate and cascades down the chakras and flows into the nadis or meridian system. How much life force you allow to flow through this closed, circular meridian system determines the size of your aura. The less blocked your chakras and meridians are, the more that energy can flow, the more voltage will be created, and the stronger your aura will be.

Small-mindedness and fear constrict your aura by creating blockages in your meridian system and closing down the tenth gate. The purpose of banis, yoga and meditation is to create enough psychic heat to integrate any limited, unbalanced concepts that you have about yourself or about life, so that you can have a greater flow of prana through your system. This creates a larger magnetic field, a stronger aura, and consequently more protection.

No one is more protective than a mother with her child. She has such auric sensitivity that when her baby is in another room and makes the smallest sound, she feels it and gets up to take care of the child's needs. The seventh month is July and astrologically the month of Cancer, which represents the mother and the aura, the seventh body. The recitation of the "Puta Mata Ki Asis" shabad eleven times a day creates a strong seventh body.

The seventh body corresponds to the pineal gland, which yogis call the tenth gate. When your pineal gland starts to radiate, you realize that you are a self-contained being who can integrate socially and also maintain a strong sense of self. You are able to deflect people's negativity and maintain your inner harmony. In the physical body, the seventh chakra rules the immune system. In Chinese medicine it corresponds to the spleen-pancreas meridian. Your immune system fights off disease the way a strong aura fights off negativity.

When your seventh body is strong, it is easy to maintain your own identity in large groups. You are equally comfortable alone or in a crowd. People who have weak auras tend to avoid crowds. With a strong aura it is easy to distinguish what thoughts are yours and what thoughts you are picking up from other people. Someone whose aura is solid can easily answer questions. The questions beam up to the aura, the aura starts to integrate them into the psyche, and then the natural flow of the intuition will move. Frequently people walk out of our yoga classes saying that the teachings during the class answered the questions they had come into class with. This is not magic, it is the result of an effective 7th body.

You typically find that someone with a strong aura is heart-centered, giving, and open with their feelings. They can easily choose how open to be with their feelings and who to be open with.

Most people do not have much aura development, which results in not experiencing a solid inner security. Then they spend their energy trying to get their security from how many cars, houses, friends or boats they have. They are trying to create security externally when it can only come from the experience of an efficient seventh body.

What is someone like when they have a weak seventh body? They look and feel scared and insecure. They are easily victimized. They maintain no sense of self-identity; they cannot maintain who they are. They are like chameleons; they will act one way around certain people and with a different group they will flip into another mode. With a weak seventh body they are easily influenced by others. Someone will say, "Let's do this," and they will do it, even if it goes against their principles.

As a chiropractor I often see insecurity expressed as lower back pain. If you have a weak aura, you might also have an inability to experience love; you might have a tight diaphragm because you are trying to protect your heart center. The yogic answer to this is to strengthen your

43

aura so that this energetic shield will protect your heart center. Then you are able to release the protective armoring around your heart center. Some physical problems that could accompany a weak seventh body are diabetes, hypoglycemia, and immune system weakness.

A strong seventh body is the key to develop your eighth, ninth, and tenth bodies. Once your aura is strong, the eighth body, the pranic body, can move more prana into the self-contained system of the aura, which then can continue to expand. Once your aura expands to a certain point, your ninth and tenth bodies, the subtle and radiant bodies, continue to expand. When that happens, your pineal gland radiates which then neutralizes external and internal negativity. You become a self-protected, organic sphere that maintains its integrity. This all starts to happen only when the seventh body, the aura, has been sufficiently developed.

Many techniques to develop the seventh body are outlined in our first book, *Numerology for Self Mastery* and you also can find other yoga and meditation kriyas to create a strong aura in the KRI kundalini yoga manuals. Yellow, sweet foods are also good for your seventh body: peaches, papayas, pineapples, and bananas. Yellow stones like citrine and amber strengthen this body. Since the pineal gland reflects the seventh body, any kind of meditation for the tenth gate will strengthen the aura. In fact, meditation is the single most effective tool you have to strengthen your seventh body.

With a strong aura your heart center can open up and blossom. This creates the feeling of security no matter what the external circumstances are. An effective seventh body will let you leap out into infinity and feel, "I am a soul! I am a self-contained, organic being in this energy field. I can isolate all the negativity around me and neutralize all my inner negativity." Once you can do that, you will be ready to experience other subtler planes of existence within your own consciousness. Then you can bring all that vastness back through the sixth center and integrate infinity into your life.

"The healing touch which God has given to a woman is unbelievably strong. You must understand, woman is the only creative creature, which God has made whose aura can become a beam. Men's auras can't do that. When a woman meditates and prays, her aura becomes a beam of light. The female aura has the power to become a beam." -

-Yogi Bhajan 1984

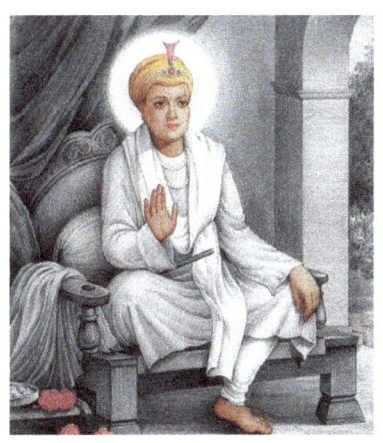

8
The Eighth Body
Archetype: Guru Har Krishan
Pranic Body
Energy, Courage, Self-Initiation

Guru Har Krishan became the Guru at the age of five, in 1661. The Hindu pundits were skeptical that a five-year-old boy was qualified to be a Guru, so they brought scholars to test him. The scholars asked Har Krishan to translate some complicated passages from the Bhagavad Gita. Nearby stood a very humble illiterate man named Chajju, who was serving water in the Guru's kitchen. The Guru reached out and tapped Chajju gently, asking him to reply to the scholars' questions. To their amazement, Chajju began to explain the passages from the Bhagavad Gita and also quote verses from the Vedas and the Upanishads. The Pandits' doubts dissolved and they bowed in humility and reverence.

In 1664 there was a smallpox epidemic in Delhi. Guru Har Krishan served water from his well to those suffering and dying. To this day the water from this same well, now at Bangla Sahib Gurdwara in Delhi, is distributed to all who come for healing. Guru Har Krishan died of smallpox at the age of 8. His life demonstrated that it is not the life that matters it is the courage that you bring to it. His last words spoke to the impermanence of the physical body and that peace is experienced when we flow with God's will.

The gift of a strong eighth body, the pranic Body, is that you experience with your every breath that you are one with the universe. By mastering your eighth body as illuminated by Guru Har Krishan, you will continuously:

- **Feel energetic**
- **Balance the three aspects of your mind**
- **Experience life from your heart**
- **Live life as an expression of love**
- **Feel courageous**

Your seventh and eighth bodies work together to transform fear into courage. Your aura provides the protective container so that prana can build up. This increasing level of prana further strengthens your aura and lets you feel even more protected and whole. This experience relaxes you and your breath even more deeply, which then transfers more prana into your aura. Your aura gets stronger and you feel more safe and alive; your heart opens and expands and fills you with love. It is a beautiful, infinite, upward spiral.

To open up your pranic body, you need to release the protective armoring around your heart so that you can breathe deeply and absorb not just more oxygen but also more prana. Oxygen is necessary for the body and prana energizes the kundalini. In order for you to release the protective armoring, your seventh body needs to be strong. Your aura must be there to protect you so that when your diaphragm and armoring start to release, you will not feel vulnerable and shut back down. Ninety-five percent of people are chest breathers; they do not breathe from the diaphragm because they are so tight from the armor, the defensive shielding, they have built up. I work with athletes, and even most of them are chest breathers. They rarely do diaphragmatic breathing. We breathe shallowly as a defense mechanism to protect our heart, by making it inaccessible. By learning how to strengthen the pranic body, we find a more enlightened and healthy way to support our heart.

Someone who knows how to read palms will find that the secondary lifeline is solid in people who have strong pranic bodies. They have a lot of reserve energy because the pranic body allows them to store reserve energy in the kidneys. Someone whose pranic body works well will not be impulsive. When someone is impulsive and premature, whether in decision-making or when intimate or with sports, it means that they can't hold energy well because they have a weak eighth body. When you can hold prana, you cherish the events in life and are not so quick to let them slip away.

Someone whose eighth body is strong is totally courageous. Yet they may be courageous without finesse. Maybe they are daredevil surfers or daredevil rock climbers. They unleash their eighth body energy in its raw form. They do not necessarily have grace yet - that comes with the development of the ninth and tenth bodies.

A weak eighth body could manifest as adrenal symptoms and conditions of fatigue and exhaustion. When someone has chronic fatigue syndrome, the diaphragm is usually shut down. They are so protective of their heart center that they won't let any energy flow. In Chinese medicine this is called a kidney deficiency. All the Chi energy generated from breathing gets stored in the kidneys, the seat of life. When you are not generating any Chi because your diaphragm is so constricted that you are barely breathing; there is nothing to put in storage.

Yogis say that the start for disease is in the malfunctioning of the pranic body. Disease occurs when prana is blocked from flowing freely through the system. The key to all healing is to bring awareness to whatever is causing the blockage so that the energy flow can be reestablished. Do whatever you can to allow that energy to flow - a vigorous yoga set or some powerful pranayam. By doing this you will see where your psyche is stuck, because when you force energy through a closed system, the weakest link gets exposed. Whenever your energy gets blocked, be with it. Hear what your psyche is telling you. Say to yourself, "I am integrating this now!" Then consciously sit down, and instead of saying, "I have got to get rid of all my neuroses," just say, "I am awesome just as I am. The heat from this pranayam is integrating all experiences. I am totally exalted."

You attain mastery of your eighth body when you become conscious of your breath and learn how to slow down your rate of breathing. The more oxygen you can take in at a very slow rate, the more mastery you have of your eighth center. Most meditations use some kind of special breath. In Kundalini Yoga the most powerful breath to activate the eight body is the 'one minute breath". Activities that encourage diaphragmatic breathing, such as aerobic exercise or chanting, also help open the pranic body.

Breath of fire is an effective tool for charging up the pranic body. This yogic breath is a balanced breath and will not increase the fire element, instead it generates the psychic heat (fire) necessary to create a harmonious flow of prana in all the bodies. Moving back and forth from camel pose into baby pose is effective in opening up the front and back of the diaphragm area, and therefore the heart center. First do them with easy, deep breathing, and then after you have opened up a little, you can continue the asana with breath of fire. Nauli Kriya done for three to five minutes first thing in the morning can loosen up the diaphragm area so that your breathing will be deeper and smoother.

Acupuncture combined with yogic breathing focused on releasing the diaphragm is effective in working with the eighth body. You have to release the diaphragm and change the breathing pattern to unblock the heart center. This is what allows prana to flow. As a chiropractor, I see eighth body problems manifest as tightness in the middle back. When I adjust that area it opens the capacity for deeper breathing.

People often live day-to-day, hand-to-mouth. Very few people are even consciously aware that they have a presence and a magnetic field. It is very difficult to develop past the seventh center. Once you create a connection with the eighth body, you must self-initiate. You self-initiate when you become conscious of an unconscious human function: the breath. Control of the breath gives you the capacity to integrate your life experiences, and this is what gives dominion over your mind. And once your mind is contained, it can reflect the light of your soul. Imagine that the mind is a lake and the soul is the bottom of the lake; if the mind is not still it will create so many waves that it becomes impossible to see the soul. This is what it means to contain the mind; you make it still so that it can do its actual job, which is to reflect the light of the soul. With a strong eighth body you are self-contained, self-fulfilled, self-illumined, self-recognized in self-ecstasy.

Everywhere you are supposed to find Guru. But in Japji you find the words 'pavan guru'. Vahan means that on which you ride. Pavan means praan – on which the praan rides. That is air. Air is the source of prana. Pavan Guru – that on which the prana rides is your Guru. When prana rides, what happens? You speak. The pranic projection between a human and a human is communication.

- Yogi Bhajan 1985

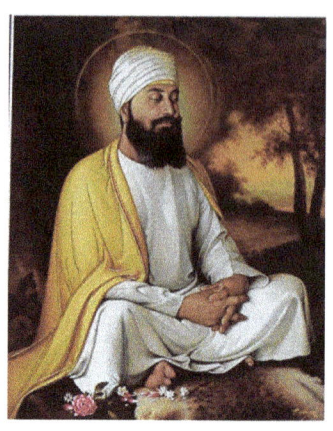

9
The Ninth Body
Archetype: Guru Teg Behadur
Subtle Body
Subtlety, Calmness, Mastery

Guru Teg Bahadur was born in 1621. He became Guru after a long selection process following Guru Har Krishan's death. Guru Har Krishan didn't appoint his successor before he died, but on his death bed he said, "Baba Bakale," meaning that that the next Guru would be found in the village of Bakale.

Makhan Shah was a wealthy sea merchant who had been a student of Guru Har Krishan. After the Guru died, Makhan Shah was at sea and a big storm came up, threatening to destroy his ship. He prayed, "Dear Guru, whoever the next Guru is, I will give you 500 gold coins if you save me and my ship." The seas calmed and the merchant was able to return safely to shore.

Makhan Shah heard that the next Guru would be found in Bakale, but when he got there he found 22 claimants to the throne, each one saying he was the next embodiment of Nanak. Makhan Shah was very confused by this, but mindful of his promise to give 500 gold coins to the Guru, he went from claimant to claimant, paying his respects and giving each one 25 gold coins. When he had finished making his rounds he asked if there was anyone else he should see. He was told, "There is

a man called Teg Bahadur. He has been meditating for 20 years."
Makhan Shah went to Teg Bahadur's house to pay his respects. But when he made his offering of 25 gold coins, the holy man came out of his meditation, opened his eyes and said, "When your ship was floundering, you promised me 500 coins. Now are you settling with 25?" Teg Bahadur showed Makhan Shan his shoulder: "You see, the wound on my shoulder has not yet healed. I carried your ship on my shoulder. Have you already forgotten your promise? Makhan Shah was overjoyed to find the real Guru. He gladly gave him 500 coins and went into town to proclaim that the Guru had been found.

During the late seventeenth century, the fanatical Muslim emperor, Jahangir, was waging a bloody campaign to convert everyone in his kingdom to Islam. The Hindu pandits came to Guru Teg Bahadur and asked for his help in withstanding the emperor's aggression. The Guru told the pandits to carry a message to the emperor that if he could convert Guru Teg Bahadur to Islam, then all Hindus would also convert. But Jahangir was unable to overcome the Guru's spiritual strength. Enraged by his failure to do so, he had Guru Teg Bahadur beheaded in 1675.

The ninth body is the subtle body. When the subtle body is strong as embodied by Guru Teg Behadur, you can see past the literal, obvious and mundane to the universal play that is manifesting. Things that used to seem mysterious or random to you start fitting into a vast pattern. It is like this: if an artist painted a huge design on a wall and then covered it up with a big thick cloth, except for one corner, it would probably be impossible for you to figure out the whole design from just the one corner you could see. That is what normal consciousness is like. You just see bits and pieces of universal reality, so you are likely to draw incomplete conclusions about what things mean, or how things fit together, or where things are going.

When your subtle body is activated, all of a sudden it is as if you have x-ray vision and you can see right through that thick cloth; you can see the whole design underneath it. You can see exactly how that corner fits into the whole design; you can see how that corner is perfect just the way it is and just where it is. This is the state of consciousness where there is no mystery; instead, there is mastery. Mastery gives you patience and calmness. You are able to see how the play of the universe is working and you play your part, letting things unfold in their own time. You have a deep understanding that things are meant to be and that there is a flow.

Where there is mastery there is no mystery. People demonstrate mastery in all areas of life. I often think of it in terms of a fine jewelry maker or craft person. When they allow their subtle body to guide them, their work will be truly refined, truly sublime.

A well-developed subtle body lets you learn things fast. It gives you conscious access to the organic, universal intelligence within you. All you have to do is focus to realize it. You can dive into any new situation and learn both the basics and the subtleties right away. You start out at a job, learn it quickly, and wind up teaching it to others. Then you are ready to go to the next level and learn that set of skills. However, people who master things quickly can also get bored easily. They will get to a certain point and then they are ready to move on because there is nothing left for them to master.

When your ninth body is well developed, you know what is underneath the surface of what people say. You can read body language and the subtleties of nonverbal communication. When someone walks into the room, you sense and observe the unconscious patterns hidden by their conscious projection. You have the capacity to recognize that most things do not need to be handled with force, and trust the unfolding that you are witnessing.

In my early days as a healer I would intuitively know something and just blurt it out. But as my subtle body became more developed, I realized that there is a time and a place for everything. The subtle body gives you the ability to trust the process of life, which gives you finesse and with that finesse you can refine your timing.

The ninth body rules the small intestine, which is part of the digestive system. Someone with a weak ninth body may have problems digesting their food. They may also have a hard time digesting and assimilating information, situations, or input of any kind. They are so critical and overly analytical that they may have a hard time letting things do what they are supposed to do. They may be restless, and lack the calmness of a well-developed subtle body because they are not at peace with the flow of the way things are.

Someone who does not have mastery is stuck in the mystery. They can be completely naïve and obtuse in the most obvious situations. When I want to evaluate myself, I stand before the mirror and run through my 10 bodies really fast - 1,2,3,4,5,6,7,8,9,10 - to see how they are doing. To test my ninth body, I close my eyes and feel the energy between my hands while concentrating on my third eye. Is my ninth body strong enough today to feel something as subtle as the energy between my hands? Or not? If it is not as strong as I want it to be, then I do something to strengthen it. It could be something as simple as putting on my nicest pair of shoes or jewelry.

When I first started doing yoga, I went to hear Yogi Bhajan give a lecture. He spoke about how to make changes in your life - do something new for forty days and you begin to break the old habits; do it for ninety days and the new habit starts to get into your subconscious; do it for one hundred and twenty days and the new habit is locked in as a part of your new behavior pattern. Then Yogi Bhajan looked right at me and said, do it for one thousand days, and you will be a master. To experience the mastery of a strong ninth body do a meditation or specific yoga kriya for one thousand days in a row.

If you are going to do something for a thousand days, have an intention. Plan it, visualize it, and be clear about what it is going to feel like when you reach it. I once talked to a man who had been meditating three hours a day for twenty years. He told me, "It has not worked." I was shocked; I could not believe someone would say he had meditated for that much time and that it didn't work. So I asked him, "Do you have an intention for doing your meditation? Did you have an idea of what you were wanting to accomplish, what you were going to feel like, and how you were going to act differently after you have done the meditation?" He said, "No, I just did it."

Yogis identified that the way energy manifests occurs in four consecutive phases - a beautiful cycle of ever expanding energy.

The four aspects in our example for a 1000 day meditation:

1. A clear **intention** for doing the meditation
2. Engage your **passion,** your mood, to align with this intention
3. **Practice** of the technology in a dedicated space
4. **Confirmation** that you are achieving the intended result

If you don't do any one of these four aspects of this Purushartha Cycle, you may be the one who says it didn't work. Follow these 4 steps above and self–fulfillment is more likely to be achieved.

I have met many people on the spiritual path who rely completely on bhakti, devotion. Devotion is an important spiritual quality especially during the Piscean age, an age that was about faith and sacrifice. Now that we are in the Aquarian age, faith needs to be integrated with experience. You need to experience the truth, not just believe it or trust what someone else says about it. The kriyas in Kundalini Yoga generate integration between bhakti and shakti energy. When you consciously practice with devotion (bhakti) and have a clear intention (shakti), you can channel outside pressure to elevate yourself and it will not stress you out.

Meditation is a tool and you have to understand what it is you are trying to accomplish with the tool. I once heard a story about a guy who showed up in the court of God and told God that he had meditated six hours a day, every day of his life, for over sixty years. God told him, "You just did the technology that is why you never found me!" The man had gone through the yoga exercises and mudras and mantras, but he had never had the projection of what he wanted to experience from doing his meditation. A lot of people think that meditating automatically brings certain results. Meditation gives you the opportunity to change your experience about the universe, it can allow you to be the master of your own God realization. It lets your universe get bigger and have more possibilities. You have to consciously have the devotion and projection of what you want your life to be.

Another gift of a strong ninth body is the ability for self-initiation. Once I talked to a lady who meditated at least three hours a day for twelve years. She dressed like a yogi and had a healthy diet; she basically did all the practices of a yogi. I asked her, "Have you sat down and acknowledged to yourself that you are a yogi?" She said, "Well not really." So I said, "How much more practice are you going to need before you are willing to make that declaration?" Self-initiation is just that: *self* -initiation. Only you can do this, and only you can recognize it when you have it.

When I started on my spiritual path I wanted to be a realized being, a yogi. At some point I observed that I had not really defined this for myself. How would I recognize it when I was realized? It is like saying, "I want to go to New York," but not know where New York is or what it looks like. So you just get in your car and drive and you end up in Philadelphia instead. If you are going somewhere, you need to know where it is and how to recognize it when you get there. Well, New York is hard to miss because the first thing you see on the road is the George Washington Bridge. Then you will see a sign that says "New York." That is how you will know you are there. If you do not know this, you could end up in Philadelphia, or Cincinnati, or Dallas, and you waste your time and energy. So use the technology of meditation and yoga to move yourself from mystery to self-mastery and claim your self-realization.

An effective ninth body expresses as self-mastery and calmness because you understand the subtleties of life. Master your ten bodies by mastering the qualities of the ten Gurus to reach your own infinity.

"Yes, gur is that basic formula. What is Guru Ram Das? People do not know. Guru Ram Das is a consolidated, saturated stage of Bhaktee, from which the power of shaktee rises. After Guru Ram Das, which Guru came? Guru Arjan. Fire purifies everything. He stood the test of purity. In shastar they call it: agan pursha, the test of fire. The light in Guru Ram Das produced Arjan, who could go through the test of fire and come out clean. Then came Guru Hargobind, miree and piree, temporal and secular: spiritual and temporal union of the power in the combined self of one being. And who came next? Guru Har Rai, kindness and mercy. He was very merciful. Then came Guru Harikrishan. Compassion, young, innocent, raw, beautiful, compassion. Then came Guru Teg

Behadur. He who takes away the pain of all. Then came who? Guru Gobind Singh. The seeker and sought after, became one. You have to look at these Gurus as part of you. Each one is you."

- *Yogi Bhajan 1983*

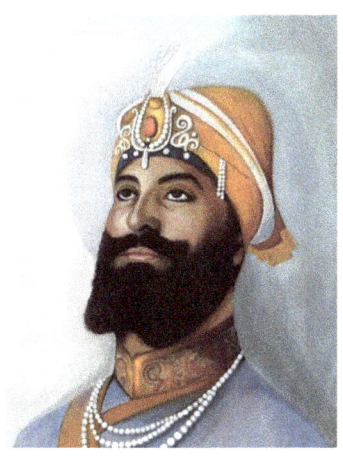

10
Tenth Body
Radiant Body
Royal Courage, Nobility, Radiance

Gobind Rai was born in 1666, the son of Guru Teg Bahadur. He exhibited great courage and elevated consciousness at a young age – when he was nine years old he advised his father to choose martyrdom. Later in life he sacrificed his own four sons so that others could maintain their freedom of consciousness. As Guru, he united the Sikhs into a community of 'Khalsa,' which means 'pure ones."

Throughout his life Guru Gobind Singh taught the sacredness of a householder's lifestyle and encouraged Sikhs to work hard, give to others, and defend the weak. He was a tireless social reformer: he raised the status of women and recruited the lower classes into his army, transforming them into courageous soldiers. Guru Gobind Singh had a versatile and charismatic personality. He was the embodiment of love and taught that those who love humanity, love God. He was a poet and a scholar, composing his works in a variety of Indian languages, including Persian and Sanskrit.

Guru Gobind Singh's teachings of love and kindness extended even to those who would seem to be his enemies. When he was compelled to take a soldier's life in battle, he would use a gold-tipped arrow so that the man's family would not be left destitute. One evening after battle, one of Guru Gobind Singh's Sikhs, Bhai Khanaiya, went to the enemy's camp and cared for the wounded soldiers. When his fellow Sikh soldiers realized what he was doing they were shocked. They went to the Guru and complained, so the Guru asked that the man be brought to him. Bhai Khanaiya answered the Guru's summons and stood before him and said: "Guru whenever I see someone in pain, I see your face in his. I no longer know who is my enemy and who is my friend." Guru Gobind Singh handed Bhai Singh some salve and said, "Put this on their wounds – they will heal even faster."

When it came time for Guru Gobind Singh to die, he wanted to liberate his Sikhs from the attachment of having a Guru in human form, so he installed the Siri Guru Granth Sahib as the eleventh and final Guru. He told his Sikhs, "Whenever you want an answer to your questions or whenever you want to be with your Guru, just read from the Siri Guru Granth Sahib or sit in its presence. The Word of God is your Guru." Guru Gobind Singh left his body in 1708.

Imagine your whole being surrounded by a glorious, radiant nine foot sphere of energy with brilliant rays of light at the outer edge of the sphere. These rays are golden, which create a visible brilliance, and cause your aura to be impenetrable. No outer negativity can enter and all inner negativity is neutralized by it. Your tenth body, the radiant body, are these rays which project out from the edge of your aura. A powerful pranayam practice connects these beams of light to the universal magnetic field. Then the energy shines and pulses, expanding the radiant beams to their maximum.

When you have a strong radiant body, you project royalty and grace. You carry yourself regally, dress well, adorn yourself with refined jewelry, and surround yourself with a beautiful, harmonious environment. Even your mannerisms express nobility: your facial expressions, your body language, and the tone and inflection of your voice. You exert a magnetic presence. When you enter a room, everyone's attention is unconsciously drawn in your direction.

Many cultures associate negative traits with the concept of royalty, which is the expression of the tenth body. In America, we value democracy and hard work. We are afraid that people with a lot of power and wealth will abuse their positions as they so often have, so we shy away from that part of ourselves, our own inner royalty. There is also an aversion to wealth in societies based on religious principles, which draw a sharp distinction between spirit and matter. Where you feel that you have to choose between either being spiritual, or enjoying life and the gifts of earthly existence. The radiant body can also be a challenge in the New Age community, which places a high value on social equality and simplicity. We are coming into the realization that, in fact, abundance, prosperity, and royalty are the basic expansive expression of our universe. It is time for us to claim our birthright in this new age and experience total abundance with consciousness.

You do not want to get into an argument with someone who has a strong radiant body because you will not win. They have so much stamina that they will never give up. These people tend to be fervent and outspoken.

The ultimate spiritual expression of the tenth body is royal courage - fearlessness with finesse. There is an artistic bent to it, a sophistication. On the football field, a guy with a strong eighth body will be fearless and robust, running as fast as he can, bashing into people. A player with a strong radiant body won't bash, he will run, then step to the right, then twist around, and run again; finesse and effortless action.

I have observed that when someone's tenth body is working they will put 110% into whatever they are doing. They give more than what is required. I have a friend like that, everything she does has a light to it. There is a certain strength you pick up when you are around her. It takes courage to give something your all, to put your entire spirit, your entire being behind what you do. The tenth body is called "all or nothing." Someone with a strong radiant body gives all, or nothing.

When a person has developed their tenth body, you will either love them or hate them. You will love them for all the light flowing through them, or you will hate them because that light exposes all your shadows. It is very difficult for people to be neutral to someone with a strong radiant body. People whose radiant bodies are developed their presence automatically causes other people to change.

Someone who is not using their tenth body can be a real "banana spine." They won't be able to confront situations in life because they have so much fear of conflict, so much fear of recognition. One way to evaluate your own radiant body is to have a conversation with yourself:

> "If I could afford to wear expensive clothing and jewelry, would I?"
> "No, I would still just wear jeans and sneakers. I don't really like standing out that much."

With a strong radiant body, you can handle all the attention you attract. A lot of people do not like that, so they dress down, act low-key, and diminish their capabilities. This popular quote from Marianne Williamson, describes the experience of a strong tenth body:

> "Our deepest fear is that we are powerful beyond measure.
> It is our light, not our darkness that most frightens us.
> And as we let our own light shine, we unconsciously give other people permission to do the same. As we are liberated from our own fear, our presence automatically liberates others."

Our favorite way of to develop the tenth body is Archer Pose. Hold this asana for eleven minutes on each side to expand your radiant body. Wearing white increases the power of your radiant body, as well as growing your hair. Reciting Guru Gobind Singh mantras and bani will activate your tenth body.

The tenth body is also called "one plus." It is one, the soul, plus your radiance. The tenth body is a state where you completely exhibit your soulful self externally. You recognize and realize your own magnificence and you can express it to others. Your divine self is so crystal clear that everyone sees it. My light is thy light. Whatever flows through me is pure radiance.

"When the mind comes out of duality, prosperity is there. The 25th paurie of Jap Ji has the power to take away duality, because it covers every aspect of the projection of the self and it's radiance. It also works on the 10th body, the radiant body, that is how prosperity is produced." **- Yogi Bhajan 1984**

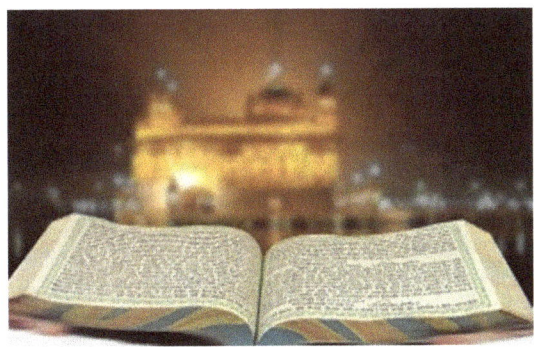

11
The Eleventh Embodiment
Archetype: Siri Guru Granth Sahib
Command Center, Completion, Flexibility

"Siri Guru Granth Sahib does not direct you. It directs your mind and you have to have control over your mind – your negative, positive and neutral mind. The trinity of mind should be under your control. The method to control the trinity of the mind is called the Yoga of Awareness, Kundalini Yoga"   **- Yogic Bhajan 1980**

The Siri Guru Granth Sahib contains the vibratory frequency of Truth. It is a living Guru for those who long to relate to the essence of their soul. The structure of the Siri Guru Granth is based on ragas, specific vibrations which direct the mind. When you read these distinct words they generate the vibrational pattern of Infinity. This Guru does not hold a philosophical discussion, instead it offers us an experience of Oneness, kindness, and love.

Let's review the ten body process to see how this 11th embodiment functions as the command center for all ten bodies. The human psyche develops slowly through the constant balancing of the gunas at the first, second, third, fourth, fifth chakras. This is the realm where we get to integrate the polarities, our karmic lessons. Then the sixth and seventh bodies provide protection and projection and the eighth body brings the fuel, the prana to energize the process and then the ninth and tenth bodies provide the capacity for a deep awareness of the subtle realms.

The eleventh position in yogic numerology is not a body. Rather, it is the completion point, the command center. It is the vantage point from which you direct the play of the ten bodies unto infinity. You realize that you are a visitor here on Earth, and that you are here to express mastery, through a continual process of self-initiation. Whatever challenges you face in life, it does not throw you off. Instead of reacting, you respond consciously from a lived experience of your Sat Nam. It is not about being perfect and never getting swayed by the polarities of the human experience, instead with a strong connection to the 11th embodiment, you notice the discordance immediately and can make the choice to respond consciously vs. react from your triggered state.

Imagine what it would be like to have complete flexibility of your psyche because you have mastered the integrated space all of your ten bodies. When you are this proficient you can connect with someone, whatever state they are in, and then lift them up. To do that you need to be in constant recognition of the space of *'Wahe Guru'*, the bliss of the realization of infinity, because from that space you have the flexibility and adaptability to be at any frequency you choose to be. It is not necessary to chant the mantra, *'Wahe Guru'*, twenty-four hours a day. It is that you need to dwell in the capacity, the flexibility, that the command center gives and which the mantra connects you to.

In the practice of Kundalini Yoga, the eleventh embodiment is where we consciously connect to Infinity. When we study the great masters, their teachings remind us not to get lost in the mundane polarized realities of the world. Spiritual teachings help to integrate friction in our lives, because friction only comes when we perceive ourselves as separate from others and don't relate to our infinite self. It is from the space of the 11th embodiment that we can observe our reactivity to the polarities because you are so connected to the frequency of Infinity.

One effective way to connect to the vibration of Infinity is to chant shabad of the Siri Guru Granth Sahib. When you chant shabad you harmonize with the frequency of Infinity and your experience of life flows from a state of Oneness.

The essential focus is your consciousness, your awareness, not your behavior. You may need to get intense in how you speak with someone to help create a change, but you are doing it with consciousness, not out of your own emotional needs or reactivity. Before, during and afterwards you dwell in the state of *'Wahe Guru'* and can be a mirror for others.

This is why a daily sadhana (yoga practice) is encouraged, so you do not lose this state of flexibility. It brings you great peace, because you realize that you can flex into any situation, stay neutral, and uplift it. Other ways to increase the space of the 11th embodiment is to bow to Siri Guru Granth Sahib, to read in an Akand Path and to do Prakash and Sukhasan.

Many spiritual paths tell us to act through the sacred heart. However, we encourage you to participate through the heart when you can and also have the flexibility to access all those other bodies when that is what is needed. There is an art to being human, to having the kind of flexibility where it does not matter what center someone is in, you are able to go there, connect with it, and create the relationship. I have seen how a real connection allows people to stop fighting for what they feel is right, and be open to other possibilities.

A strong command from this eleventh embodiment gives you mastery of the entire physical realm and spiritual realm.

Create your Destiny with Yogic Numerology

The ten-body model of the human psyche provides an integrated, holistic approach to the experience of our humanness. Instead of looking for what is wrong pathologically and trying to fix that one thing, we see an opportunity to create a dynamic, flexible process where the goal is not simply to fix, but to integrate.

Many of the ancient cultures have circular models of reality. For example, the Native American sand paintings and the Buddhist mandalas are visual representations of a circular model of reality. In some Native American cultures, when a person exhibits a fragmented psyche, the shaman will construct an elaborate mandala of sand as a way of restoring the person to harmony. The ideograms of the *I Ching* have the same purpose. The whole technology of these ten bodies is for the purpose of re-integrating the human psyche back to its infinite wholeness.

This is where it gets to be fun! You can now choose to change your destiny by choosing a high level of awareness about your unique journey this lifetime. Your personal numerology presents the opportunity to observe how well you are using your assets and how you are working with your challenges. Remember as explained in our book: Numerology for Self Mastery:

- Your <u>assets</u> are your **destiny** and **gift** numbers
- Your <u>challenges</u> are your **karma, soul** and **path** numbers

The gift and destiny are the road you walk on; you have mastered both of these already in past life times, and they are with you to support and bring you strength for the journey. You need to include the essence of them into your life. The challenges represent the opportunities where you can actually change your destiny! Imagine a potter. She works with a clump of clay and can fashion that into any piece of art. Your challenges are your clump of clay; it's all the same stuff just not fashioned into an intentional creation. There will be pain in this process of transformation, but with this awareness to re-write your destiny, suffering becomes optional.

By observing your sensations you can measure your success with this process. If your life is a peaceful, expansive expression, then you are creating your destiny. If you are reacting, then you are in a place of hanging out with your karmic patterns and not growing. We know that energy can only increase or decrease, and that it is impossible for energy to remain stagnant. Therefore, if you are not expanding then you are contracting.

One of the most important assets to cultivate is the habit of deep listening. This is not the kind of listening where you are formulating your answer or judging if the information is true or not. By deeply listening you can learn how to evaluate yourself moment to moment: "Do I have access to all my ten bodies right now?" I used to evaluate myself once a day in the morning. Now it is an ongoing process. When I realize that one of my bodies is not engaged, I just shut my eyes and re-create a balanced space for that body so that it works again. When I meditate, I do not do it to solve problems. I just meditate on feeling my third eye opening and my tenth gate expanding. If issues come up, I do not focus on them. I just let the energy flow and let the answers come, as it is awareness which heals and integrates. We are after all human beings and not human doings!

> *Knowing your personal bodies gives you your identity.*
> *Applying all ten bodies gives you your infinity.*

When I was younger I wondered what I would be like when I was more spiritual and I thought, "I will reach a certain state and then I will be a saint. I will look like this, and feel like that, and will always stay the same." But now I see it differently. Now I see that consciousness is a state of constant flexibility, adaptability and growth where you are always experiencing newness in yourself and finding creative, expansive ways to deal with whatever comes your way.

One interpretation of the concept of 'dharma' is 'a structure to exponentially grow'. You don't reach an ultimate state and then stay the same. What it really means to be a whole, self-realized being is to be nonlinear, circular, flexible, and adaptable, to exist in a constant state of soul-oriented growth that is propelled by cosmic energy, which has no beginning, no end, no limits at all.

How do I know when my ten bodies are working? I am joyfully creative, obedient to my consciousness, and I see spirit in everyone. I evaluate the input of my mind to reach a compassionate, integrated neutral place and I have the capacity to create sacredness, to sacrifice, and to live in balance. I am intuitive and focused. I am secure and courageous. I am calm and subtle and achieve mastery. I have royal courage. I am complete and self-realized and I direct my ten bodies from an impersonal space that allows infinity to flow through me. I live in the ecstasy of my own Infinite consciousness.

This is our ten-body affirmation:

> **I am**
>
> a creative,
> connected,
> blissful,
> yogi,
> a teacher,
> who is focused,
> self contained,
> and courageous.
> I am the master
> of my own radiance
> unto infinity.

We invite you to write your affirmation based on the five positions from your numerology calculation. Each body will have its own "feel", its own "signature" and as you read the chapters on each of the numbers, one word will 'speak' to you. Use these words to create your personal numerology mantra.

SELF MASTERY

SOUL   GIFT

———   ———

                              PATH

KARMA   DESTINY

PERSONAL NUMEROLOGY HAIKU

_____

Yoga Practices to Create your Destiny

The following yoga sets and meditations are from personal notes made during yoga classes taught by Yogi Bhajan during the 1970's.

BEFORE STARTING A YOGA SET OR MEDITATION:

We recommend that you adjust the flow of your psyche to radiate, to be in tune with the universal magnetic field. In Kundalini Yoga we chant the Adi mantra: *'Ong Namo GuruDev Namo'* to create this connection. *'Ong'* can be translated as "creative consciousness" and *'Guru Dev'* means "personified light". The *"Guru"* is always external and is what guides you to your true self by using a Gur or formula for self-realization. By consciously chanting this mantra the Kundalini Yoga student sets the intention to follow the essence of the teachings, and not the personality of the teacher.

"There is no such thing as a guru within. It is a total ignorance. Guru is always without, God is always within. Guru is without; Guru is right out, Guru is the guide, Guru guides you to go within." **- Yogi Bhajan 1975**

Sit in Easy Pose with the spine straight. Put the hands together over the heart chakra in Prayer Pose. The palms are together with the fingers pointing up, pressing the thumbs into the chest, at the sternum. Inhale deeply and focus your concentration at the third eye and then chant the mantra: *'Ong Namo Guru Dev Namo'* three times.

DURING THE YOGA KRIYA (specific series of asanas)

Training the mind and the body to be in synchronicity with the breath is a critically important aspect of Kundalini Yoga as it supports you to embody this human experience. While doing the asanas, we mentally vibrate the sound *'Sat'* on the inhale and *'Nam'* on the exhale. 'Sat' means truth and 'Nam' means identity. This mantra is applied to harmonize the body, mind, and breath unless otherwise specified in the yoga set or meditation. When your mind drifts off be patient with yourself. When drifting occurs simply remember to focus and gently bring your awareness back to the breath and the mantra. Always intend to be focused, and be forgiving when that focus fades.

The following are abbreviations and other frequently used words that you will find in the descriptions of the yoga sets and meditations in this book.

Locks (Bandhas)

MB: Mulbandh is the root lock. It is a process of contracting all 3 of the following muscle groups at the same time:

- The rectal muscles
- The muscles that control the sexual organs and urination
- The navel point (pull it towards your spine).

This is done in conjunction with:

- Holding your chin in
- Lifting your heart up
- Rolling your eyes up internally and looking at the screen of your forehead
- Concentrating at your third eye

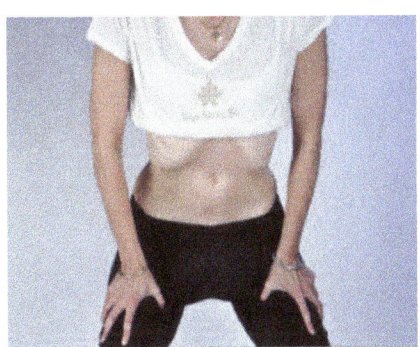

Diaphragm Lock (Uddiyana Bandh) To master this bhanda, we recommend that you include it in your daily practice. Do this with absolutely no food or liquid in your stomach. Practice it first thing in the morning after your cold shower while standing in front of a mirror. Place your hands above your knees at the tops of your thighs while bending forward slightly (30°). Exhale your breath out and do not allow any breath to come back into the lungs while applying the bhanda. With your breath held out, pull your abdominal muscles in and up. Make sure that the muscles of your diaphragm pull up and in, and then also pull up under the rib cage. The key to this is to apply pressure downward with your hands where you have placed them above your knees. Repeat holding and releasing the lock several times with your breath held out.

Neck Lock (Jalandhar Bandh) This bandha is applied during meditation, while chanting and during pranayama (the art of working with the energy of the subtle breath). It facilitates the kundalini energy to rise into the higher centers. Lift your heart as you stretch the back of your neck, keeping your head level and centered. You should feel a slight pressure at your throat.

Maha Bandh is a special lock in Kundalini Yoga that is applied in order to move the kundalini energy up through the sushmana channel, which creates a state of courage. On an exhale, apply all three bandhas: MB, neck lock and the diaphragm lock, and focus at the brow point.

These bandhas protect as they align the physical and energetic structures to allow the kundalini to rise up the central sushmana channel.

KC: Kundalini Close refers to the completion/ending of an asana. It is what you do to consolidate the projection-connection-reception of your radiant body.

At the end of an asana, inhale and hold your breath as you:

- **Focus at your third eye, between your eyebrows at the bridge of your nose**
- **Pull your chin in slightly**
- **Lift your heart center up**
- **Contract MB**

KC will conclude all asanas and meditations unless otherwise stated.

Seals (Mudras)

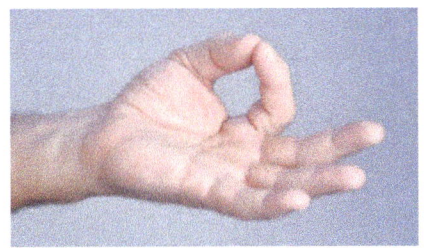

GM: Gyan Mudra. The tip of your thumb touches the tip of your index finger. This mudra gives mastery over the energy of Jupiter, the expression of expansion and knowledge. When you need more knowledge or you need expansion in your consciousness to deal with some event, then choose GM. Mastery of the mudra will give you control over the positive aspects of the planet Jupiter and it will eliminate the negative patterns that you may have picked up in this life or a past life. Incorporating this mudra into your daily practice is an effective way to align with the planetary influence of Jupiter for the benefit of your higher self.

Shuni Mudra can give you mastery over the energy of the planet Saturn. Touch the tip of your thumb to the tip of your second finger next to your index finger (middle finger). This mudra seals in the energy of Saturn and gives both wisdom and patience. Life may be showing you 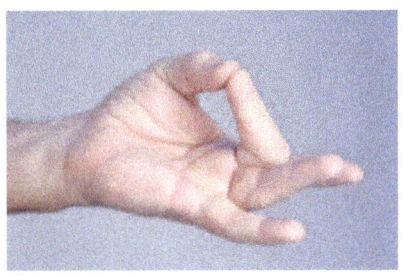 your impatience and/or a lack of wisdom in your decision making process. Always imagine Saturn's positive aspects of patience and wisdom before embarking on this journey of transforming old karmic tendencies. This alchemical process is the journey of our lifetime, our destiny work, our dharma.

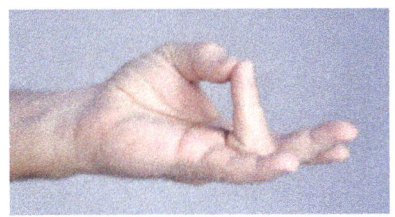

Surya Mudra is made by holding the tip of your thumb to the tip of your ring finger. This mudra seals in the energy of the Sun, and brings about physical vitality. If you feel weak and do not have the energy to show up for your life, mastering this mudra can connect you essentially with all the energy you want in order to physically handle the challenges and requirements of living your life.

Buddhi Mudra is formed by touching the tip of your thumb to the tip of your smallest finger, the pinky finger. This mudra relates to the planet Mercury and rules the aspect of communication. Mastery of this mudra reveals a 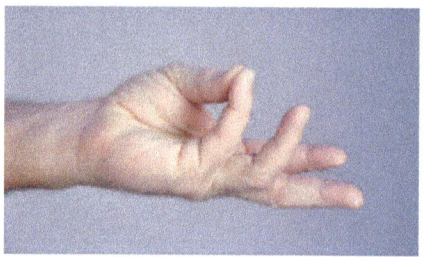 conscious relationship to communication. Communication is about effective speaking, as well as the ability to listen. If this is an area of concern, then the yogi who does this mudra with devotion will realize powerful awareness shifts in all aspects of conscious communication.

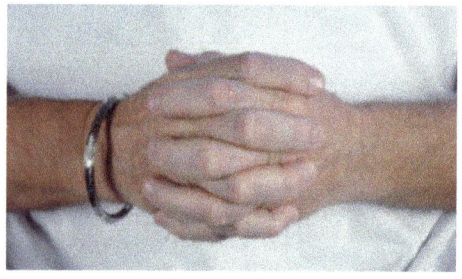 **VL: Venus Lock** masters the balance between the energies of Venus and Mars. Venus expresses the feminine energy of love and harmony and Mars expresses the masculine energies of passionate impulse and action. If you find there is too much or too little love or passion in your relationships, then conscious application of VL can transform these karmic patterns. It will create a balance between the two complimentary energies needed to achieve fulfillment in relationships. Mastery transforms negative influence and allows the positive to be summoned forth as a new, permanent habit. For those who identify with feminine energy, interlace the fingers with your right little finger on the bottom. Put your right thumb above the base of your left thumb on the webbing between your thumb and index finger. Press the tip of your left thumb on the fleshy mound at the base of your right thumb. Reverse this mudra for those who identify with masculine energy.

Pranayam (Subtle Breath)

BOF: Breath of Fire is a balancing breath generated by a rapid, continuous movement of the abdominal muscles. Practiced through your nostrils, exhale as you press the navel point back toward the spine. The inhale will come in as part of relaxation of your abdomen, rather than through effort. Sit comfortably with a straight spine. Rest your hands on your knees, palms up, with the fingers in GM, touch the tips of the index finger to the tips of the thumbs. Breathe fairly rapidly about two or three breaths per second through your nose while you pump the navel point and abdomen. Pull your abdomen in on the exhale, and relax it out during the inhale. Your chest and face should be relaxed.

When you are finished, inhale deeply and hold the breath while you pull the energy up into your higher centers. Then exhale and relax. This is a balanced breath with no emphasis on either the inhale or the exhale. Think of it as one continuous breath being pulled in and out. You will not hyperventilate if you do not breathe through your mouth.

Start practicing breath of fire for no more than 3 minutes at a time and work up to 31 minutes or more.

Once mastered, BOF can be done for a very long period of time. Yogis know that at birth each person is granted a certain amount of breaths. When Yogi Bhajan instructed us to do BOF, we were all concerned that we were using up our breaths too fast! He explained that if you do BOF unbroken, it is considered to be one breath, even if you do it for 31 minutes.

LDB: Long deep breathing. Sit in easy pose; inhale through your nose and bring as much air into your lower lungs as possible. The signature of a long deep breath is that you see your abdomen go out first as you pull the air in, then the air moves up and fills the middle of the lungs, and finally the air fills the upper part of the lungs (clavicular area).

Continue LDB in three equal parts: inhaling the air first into your lower, then to your middle, and then your upper lungs. As you exhale, release all of the air first out of the upper part of your lungs, then the middle and finally the lower, by pushing your abdomen towards your spine.

To create a complete mudra (seal) for the flow of energy, focus your eyes at the tip of your nose or at your third eye. As yogis we strive to create a habit of this natural breath and train the lungs as frequently as possible throughout the day by consciously breathing long and deep.

Common Asanas

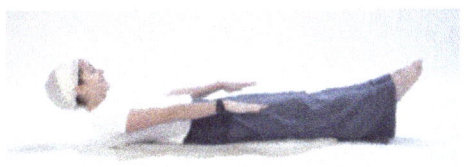

Stretch Pose: Lie on your back on a firm, cushioned surface. Stretch your legs forward with feet together and toes pointed, extend your arms parallel to your hips, but not touching them, with your fingertips pointing toward your toes, palms down. Raise your arms, feet and head 6 inches off the floor and focus your eyes on your toes. Hold this position for 1 to 3 minutes or longer, with LDB or BOF.

Sat Kriya: A fundamental kriya to Kundalini Yoga, it directly stimulates and channels the kundalini energy to move up the sushmana channel. Sit on the heels and lift your arms up with palms together. Interlace all fingers except your index fingers, which point up. Those who identify masculine, cross the right thumb over the left thumb and those who identify feminine cross the left thumb over the right. As you pull in your navel, chant "Sat" powerfully and chant "Nam" as you relax the navel. To end, inhale and apply MB, then exhale and hold your breath out as 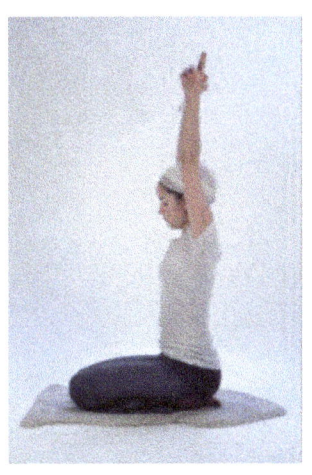 you apply Maha Bandh (all locks) and visualize the energy moving out of the tenth gate (top of your head) into the Cosmos. Inhale and relax with your forehead on the ground.

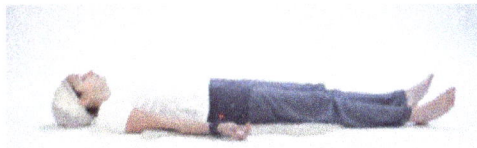

Corpse Pose: Lie on your back with your legs slightly apart, arms by your sides with palms facing up. Yoga masters often refer to this asana as a difficult pose, since it requires complete release, stillness and surrender. This is where the effects of the kriya are absorbed into the physical body and where the subtle bodies harmonize.

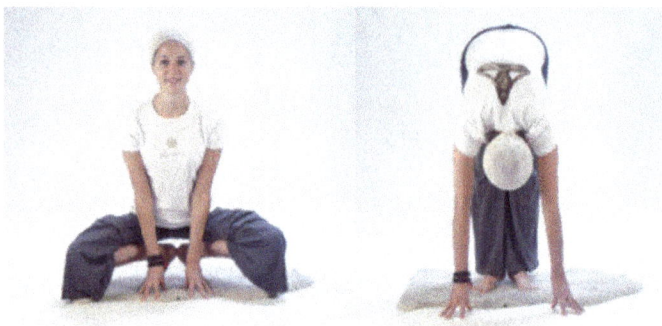

Frog Pose: Squat down, keeping your heels off the ground, and place your fingers on the ground in front of your toes. Your arms are in between your knees. Inhale, straighten your legs and keep your head down. Exhale, squatting down with your heels off the ground and lift your head so it is in line with your spine.

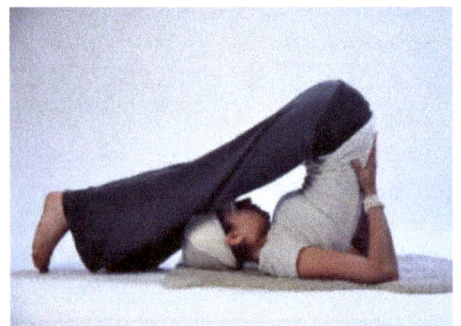

Plow Pose: Lying on your back, raise your legs up to 90° (Shoulder Stand), then continue to lift them past your shoulders until your toes touch the ground over your head. Your arms can be raised above your head with your hands holding your feet, or your arms can stay at your sides.

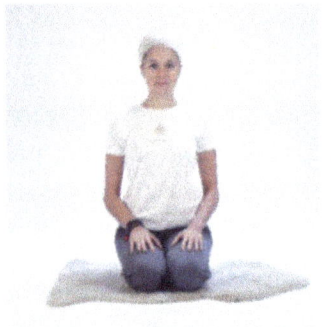

Rock Pose: Sit on your heels, mindful to keep your feet next to each other and not crossed. Your hands rest flat on your thighs with your palms face down.

Easy Pose: Sit with your legs crossed. If your knees do not come down enough to allow for a comfortable seat, then sit on a meditation pillow. This will help to bring your low back in correct alignment, which allows your hips to release and your knees to lower. This posture is often difficult for adult Westerners, as many have unlearned sitting on the floor, which keeps the hips flexible. Sitting in chairs causes the hamstrings to shorten and leads to a loss of flexibility in the hips. This self-corrects slowly as you sit on the floor and practice, practice, practice.

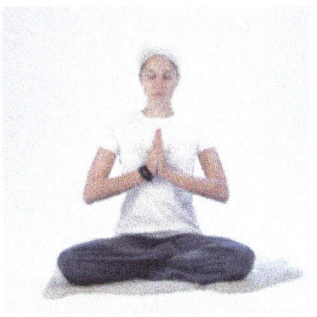

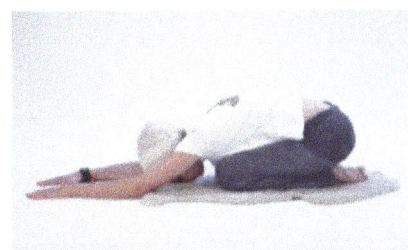

Gurpranam / Baby Pose: Sit on your heels and place your forehead on the ground in front of your knees. Your arms are by your sides, palms facing up, or your arms are straight out in front of you, palms facing down.

Mantra

ਸਤਿ ਨਾਮੁ ਕਰਤਾ ਪੁਰਖੁ ਨਿਰਭਉ ਨਿਰਵੈਰੁ

ਅਕਾਲ ਮੂਰਤਿ ਅਜੂਨੀ ਸੈਭੰ ਗੁਰ ਪ੍ਰਸਾਦਿ ॥

In Kundalini Yoga we use the "yoga of sound" often during the kriyas and meditations. Sacred sound is referred to as the 'Shabad Guru' and this is the Guru in the Kundalini Yoga lineage. There is no personality established as Guru, only the permutation and combination of specific sacred sounds. The mantras stimulate the higher glands and move the yogi's awareness from ("Gu") darkness into ("Ru") light. Mantras can be repeated 108 times per day to raise awareness of the vibratory essence of the experience of "Truth," beyond time and space, beyond right and wrong, that which always was, is, and will be.

When no other instruction is given during an asana, mentally vibrate the mantra **"Sat"** on the inhale, and **"Nam"** on the exhale. "Sat Nam" holds the mind present and attunes your personal energy to a universal frequency.

Drishti or Eye Focus

An eye focus is part of creating a mudra or energy seal during any asana or meditation as it channels the mind and causes glandular secretions when the eye muscles massage the higher glands.

Third eye point: The point between the eyebrows at the bridge of the nose. This is the default focus for any asana or meditation if no other instruction has been given. It activates the pituitary gland and balances the nervous system.

Tip of the nose: Eyes are 9/10th closed and the focus is at the tip of the nose. This focus stimulates the pituitary gland and the frontal lobe of the brain. It is very difficult for most yogis to hold this dhristi. Make it your priority to practice this important yogic skill. Look at the nose with your left eye closed and see if you can see the tip of the nose with your right eye. Then close the right eye and see if you can see the tip of the nose with the left eye. Keep practicing until you are sure you can see the tip of the nose equally with both eyes when applying this dhristi.

Chin point: Eyes are closed and internally look down at the chin, the lunar center.

Crown chakra: Located at the top of the skull. Eyes are closed and internally looking out the top of the head, stimulating the pineal gland.

End Each Yoga Kriya with this Long Deep Relaxation Routine

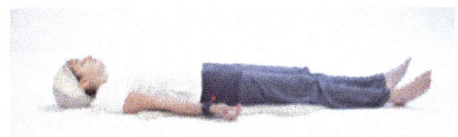

Inhale and hold your breath briefly to consolidate the energy, then as you exhale, lie on your back in corpse pose. Your arms are by your sides with your palms face-up and your legs spread 12 inches apart. You can cover yourself with a blanket and listen to a gong or other harmonic/healing sound as you deeply relax for 10 minutes.

To come out of the relaxation:

1) Deeply inhale and exhale several times, then begin to move your wrists and ankles in small circles.

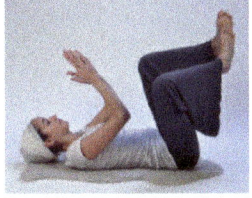

2) Rub your palms together and the soles of your feet together briskly.

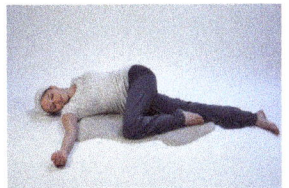

3) Keep shoulders on the floor and move the right knee up and over onto the ground to the left side of the body, repeat on other side.

4) Pull your knees to your heart center, wrap your arms around your knees and rock forward and backward on your spine several times as you inhale up and exhale down.

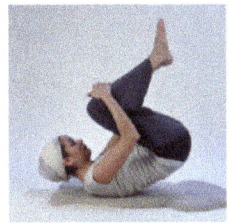

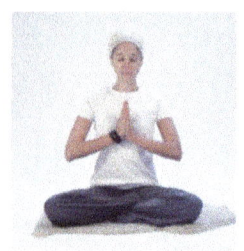

5) Sit up into easy pose with your hands in prayer pose and sing:

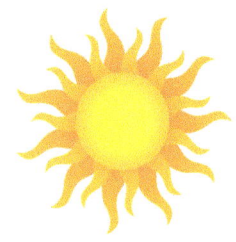

May the Long Time Sun Shine Upon You
All Love Surround You
And the Pure Light Within You
Guide Your Way On

Close the kriya by chanting one long **"*Sat Nam"***

This completes our practice, our sacred ceremony.

Medical Disclaimer

During a Kundalini Yoga class the teacher never touches the yoga student to adjust the posture, because the responsibility to "stretch" is the student's. With the same mindfulness, we ask you to do these asanas and to stop if ever there is uncomfortable pain. A teacher will inspire you to "stretch" yourself, yet as with any exercise routine, you need to build your strength and flexibility up gradually. Find a Kundalini Yoga teacher (www.3HO.com) in your area to take classes and learn the techniques and specific Kundalini Yoga practices. If you have a health condition, please consult your physician before attempting any new exercise routine. Practicing Kundalini Yoga kriyas or meditations will create fast and powerful change. It is ideal to find a certified teacher who can offer support in this change process.

First Body
Soul Body

Kundalini Yoga to Create Your Destiny
Harmonize the 1st Body
Balance the Stomach and Spleen/Pancreas Meridians

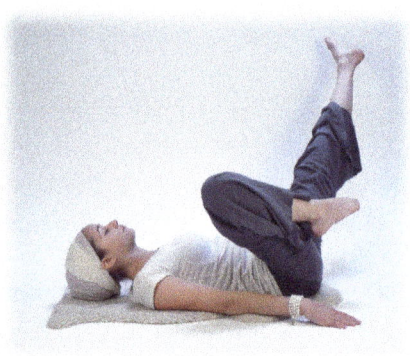

1. Lie on your back with your head flat on the ground. Bring your legs up and then spread them apart to 60º. Inhale as the left foot comes into the groin area and the right leg stays out at 60º. Exhale as the right leg comes to the groin area and your left leg moves out to 60º. Continue to move the legs in and out with the breath for **1-3 minutes**. Inhale as you hold the posture and then exhale and relax flat on the ground.

2. Sit up and spread the legs wide apart. Reach down and hold your right toes with both hands. Inhale as you move the upper torso up and then exhale as you move the chest down to the thighs. Continue with the right leg for 1½ minutes and switch and hold the left toes and repeat the asana on the left side for **1½ minutes.**

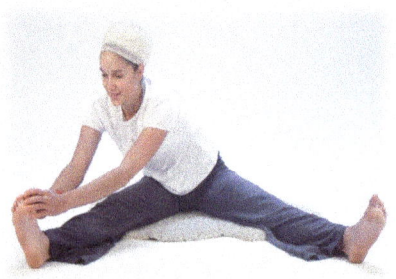

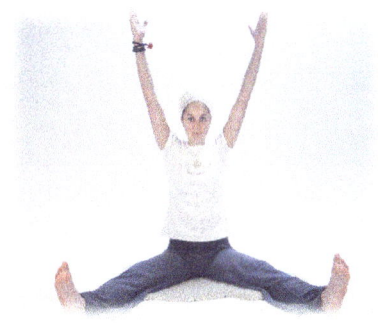

3. Continue to sit with the legs spread wide apart and raise arms up straight above the head. Inhale as you sit up straight in the center and exhale as you reach both the arms down to the left leg then inhale up to the center and exhale as you stretch both arms over to the right.

Continue this asana for **1-3 minutes.**

Sit in Easy Pose with hands in the lap for **1 minute.**

4. Sit with the left leg extended out and the right foot close into the groin. Hold the big toe with both hands, look at toe. **BOF for 1-3 minutes.** Change legs and hold the left leg with BOF for **1-3 minutes.**

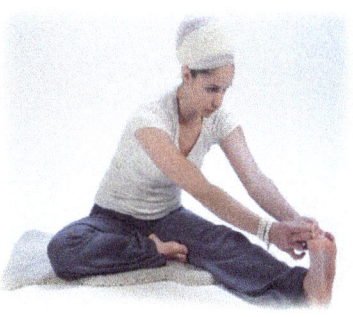

Inhale into Easy Pose and sit with the hands in the lap for **1 minute.**

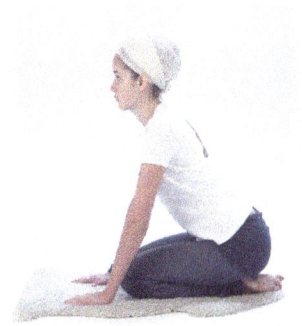

5. Sit on the heels with the hands on the floor in front of the body. In this posture do spine flex for **1-3 minutes.**

6. Sit on the heels and raise your arms up above the head in Sat Kriya position. Do Sat Kriya for **3-6 minutes.**

7. Long Deep Relaxation

Meditation to Create Your Destiny
Harmonize the 1st Body

Part 1) Sit in Easy Pose with the hands in GM on the knees.
LDB concentrating at the base of the spine for **1-3 minutes**, then LDB concentrating at the navel point for **1-3 minutes**, then LDB concentrating at the toes for **1-3 minutes**.
Sit without a focus for **1 minute**.

The body will become clean, clear and powerful.

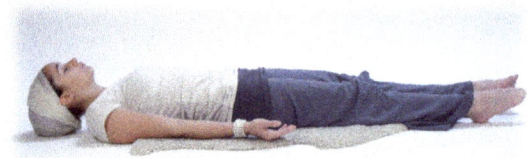

Part 2) Lie on back with hands by the sides and palms facing up. Press toes forward with strong constant pressure for **2 minutes.**

Relax in Corpse Pose for **1 minute.**

Part 3) Repeat part 2.

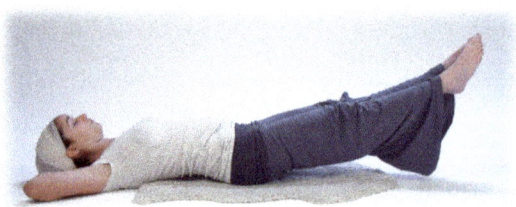

Part 4) Lie on back with hands interlaced under the neck and elbows flat against the ground. Apply a slight MB to engage the core and then lift both feet one foot off the ground with the legs straight. (You can place the hands under the hips to support your low back if needed).
LDB for **3 minutes** or until the cheeks burn.

Relax for **3 minutes** in Corpse Pose.

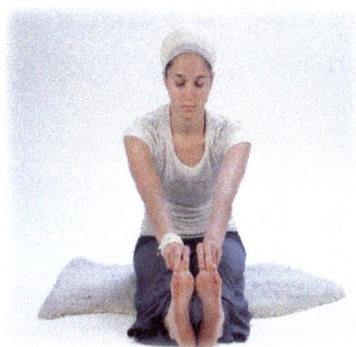

Part 5) Sit with both legs stretched out in front. Reach down and hold toes. Life Nerve Stretch: Inhale, move upper body up and exhale, move upper body down towards the thighs. Continue for **3 minutes**.

Part 6) Sit in Easy Pose with the hands resting in GM on the knees. Meditate and feel that you are the light of your soul with LDB for **11 to 31minutes**.

Eye focus is at the tip of the nose.

To End) Sing the The Long Time Sun song.

Second Body
Negative/Protective Mind

Kundalini Yoga to Create Your Destiny
Harmonize the 2nd Body
Balance the Bladder and Kidney Meridians

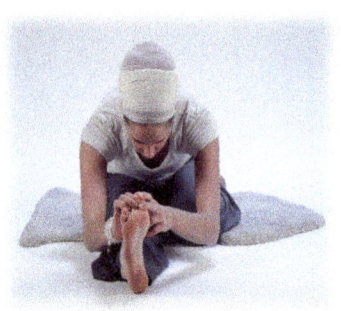

1. Sit on the left heel with the right leg extended in front. Hold the toes of the right foot with both hands. Apply MB and LDB for **1-3 minutes**.

Switch sides. Sit on right heel with the left leg extended in front. Hold the toes of the left foot with both hands. Apply MB and LDB for **1-3 minutes**.

2. Sit in Easy Pose. Hold on to the right big toe with the right hand and hold the left big toe with the left hand. Apply a slight MB to engage the core and lift into Kundalini Lotus Pose with the legs up 60º and spread wide apart. Balance on the buttocks with LDB for **3 minutes**.

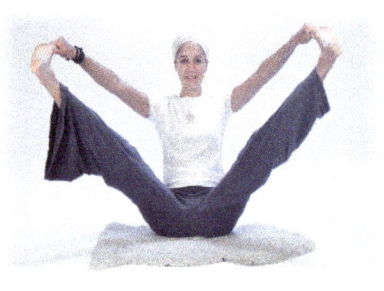

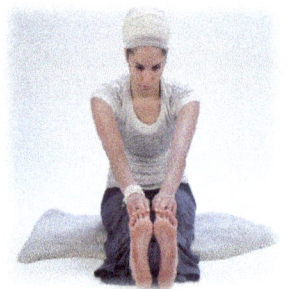

3. Sit with both legs stretched out in front of the body. Reach forward and hold the toes, keep the elbows straight. Apply MB. Stare at the big toes, pull back on the toes, hold the back straight with LDB for **1-3 minutes.**

4. Sit with the legs out straight. Place hands or elbows on the floor behind you with the fingers pointing at the toes. Lean back on your hands or raise up on elbows. Raise the 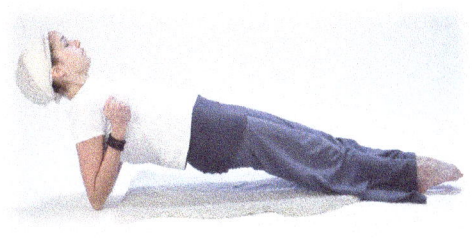 buttocks in line with the body into Back Platform Pose. Apply a slight neck lock to keep the neck in line with the body. LDB for **1-3 minutes.**

Corpse Pose for **1 minute.**

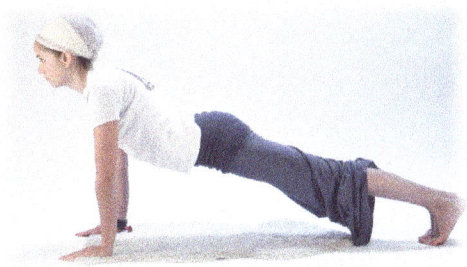 5. Chin on ground. Hands under the shoulders, spread fingers wide, raise the body either on the toes or knees and hands into Front Platform Pose.

Slowly begin doing push-ups, inhale up and exhale down. Keep a slight MB applied the entire time. **1-3 minutes.**
Lie on stomach, turn the head to one side, hands back by the hips, the palms face up. Relax **1 minute.**

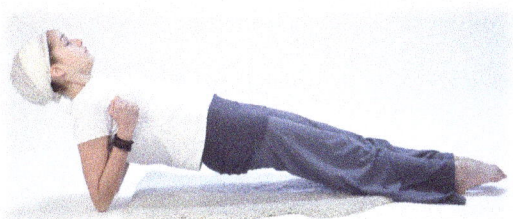

6. On back, come into a modified Back Platform Pose, on the elbows and heels. Keep the head straight. Keep MB applied with LDB. Continue for **1-3 minutes.**

Corpse Pose for **1 minute.**

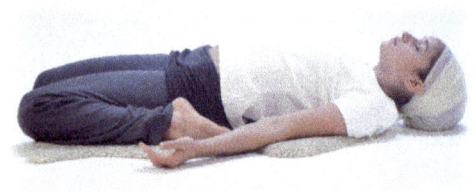

7. Sit in Rock Pose on or in between the heels and lean back all the way. LDB for **1-3 minutes.**

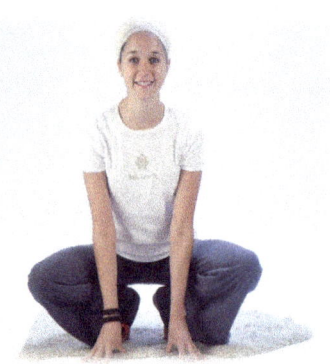
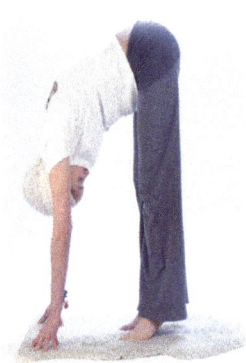

8. Stand in Frog Pose position. Do **30 frog poses**, inhale up and exhale down, keep heels off the ground.

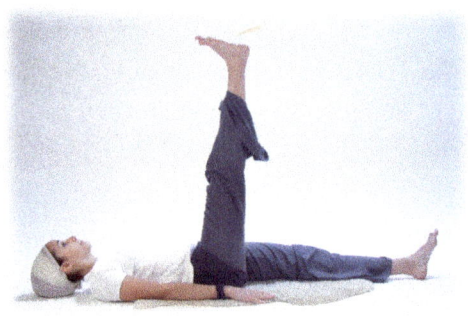

9. Lie on back, hands palms down by your hips. Inhale, left leg moves up to 90°, exhale, lower left leg down. On the next inhale, move the right leg up to 90° and exhale the right leg down. Continue alternate leg lifts for **1-3 minutes** with a slight MB.

10) Easy Pose with hands in Prayer Pose at the heart chakra, LDB. Negate all identification. I am not this body; I am not this mind, **5-7 minutes.**

11) Long Deep Relaxation

Meditation To Create Your Destiny
Harmonize the 2nd Body

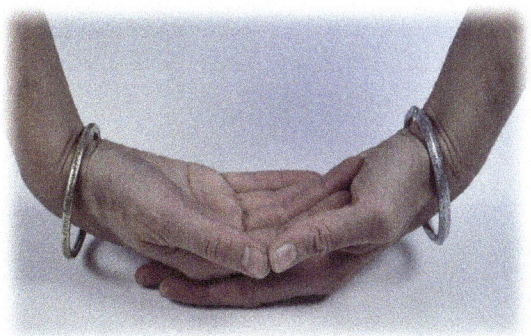

Part 1) Sit in Easy Pose, hands in the lap, thumbs touching. To increase the masculine energy place right hand on top, to increase feminine energy place the left hand on top.

Focus eyes at 3rd eye.
Chant *'Ad guray nameh, jugad guray nameh, sat guray nameh, siri guru devay nameh'* in a whisper for **11 minutes**.

Part 2) Same posture as part 1:
Chant *'Gobinday, mukanday, udharay, aparay, hariang, kariang, nirnamay, akamay'* in a whisper for **11 minutes**.

Part 3) Same posture. Chant *'SaTaNaMa Wahay Guru'* out loud, moving the head in the following way for **11 minutes:**

        SA   head straight in the middle
        TA   turn head to left
        NA   head straight
        MA   left
        WA   middle
        HAY right
        GU   middle
        RU   right

To End) Sing the Long Time Sun song.

Third Body
Positive/Projective Mind

Kundalini Yoga to Create Your Destiny
Harmonize the 3rd Body
Balance the Gallbladder and Liver Meridians

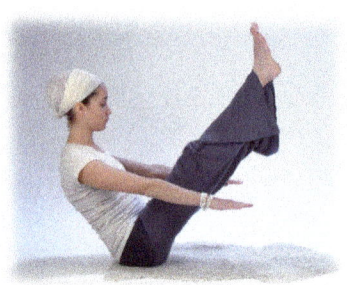

1 a. Sit with legs extended out in front and arms above the legs, palms face down and parallel to the ground. Apply a slight MB to engage the core, lean back 60° with neck in alignment with the spine as you raise the legs up to 60°, hold the arms parallel to the ground and hold Victory Pose for **60 seconds** with LDB.

1 b. Bend forward and hold toes, relax down to the thighs with LDB for **3 minutes**.

Repeat entire first exercise (1 a and 1b).

Lie on back and rest for **1 minute**.

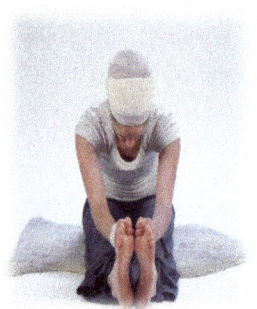

2. Rock Pose on heels and flex spine. Whisper '*Sat*' on the inhale and move the spine forward. Whisper '**Nam**' on the exhale and move the spine back. **4- 8 minutes.**

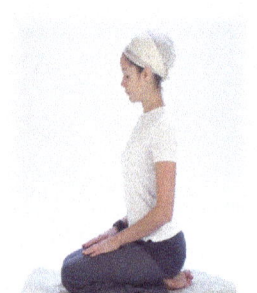
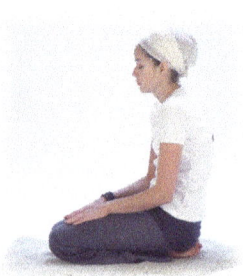

3. Sit in Easy Pose with hands in Prayer Pose at heart center. Press the entire weight into the palms with right thumb locked over the left one. Concentrate at 3rd eye with LDB. **5-10 minutes.**

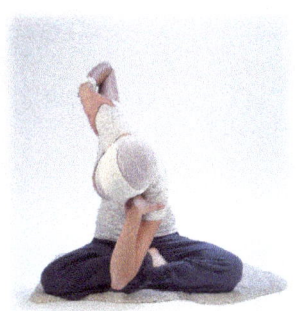

4. Easy Pose with the hands on the shoulders, fingers in front and thumbs in back. Inhale when facing straight, exhale and move the right elbow down to left knee stretching out the side, inhale and move back to center, exhale and bend to left side. Continue for **1- 3 minutes**

5. Easy Pose, hold shins. Inhale and stretch spine forward, exhale move the spine backward. Focus on accentuating the forward motion. **3 minutes.**

6. Easy Pose hands rest on knees in GM. Chant the mantra *'Sat Nam Wahe Guru'* as you move your head in the following way for **11 minutes**:

> *'Sat'*   middle
> *'Nam'*   left
> *'Wahe'* middle
> *'Guru'* right

7. Long Deep Relaxation

Meditation To Create Your Destiny
Harmonize the 3rd Body

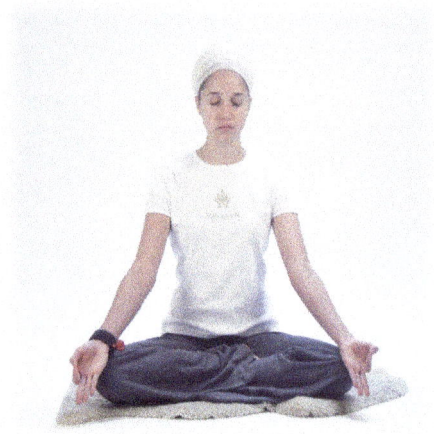

Easy Pose with hands resting on the knees in GM. Bring entire energy and consciousness to the third center at the navel point.

Silently vibrate *'Sa Ta Na Ma'* in Kirtan Kriya style moving the fingers for **11 minutes.**

Continue to chant out loud for another **5 minutes.**

Inhale, stretch the spine up and relax and project out of the body. Imagine going into the universe, keep imagining going out of the body for **5 – 11 minutes**.

Inhale and relax.

To End) Sing the Long Time Sun song.

Fourth Body
Neutral Mind

Kundalini Yoga to Create Your Destiny
Harmonize the 4th Body
Balance the Lung and Large Intestine Meridians

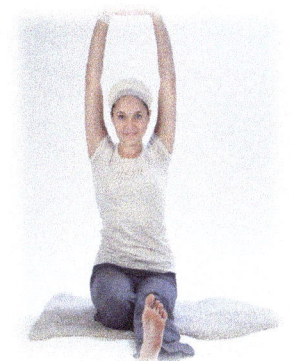

1a. Sit on right heel with left leg extended out in front. Bring both arms up with hands above head in inverted Venus Lock, palms face up. Inhale in the up position; exhale bring the chest to the left thigh with the hands reaching over the toes of left leg. Inhale up and exhale down for **3 minutes.**

To end: Inhale then exhale bring chest to left thigh and hold breath out with MB for **20 seconds.**

1b. Sit on left heel with right leg extended out in front. Bring both arms up with hands above head in inverted Venus Lock. Inhale in the up position, exhale bring chest to the right thigh with the hands reaching over the toes of right leg. Inhale up and exhale down for **3 minutes.**

To end: Inhale then exhale bring chest to right thigh and hold breath out with MB for **20 seconds.**

2. Easy Pose with hands in lap for **1 minute**.

3. Easy Pose with arms straight and hands in inverted Venus Lock raised above the head. Inhale and twist to the left, exhale and twist right.

Move rapidly for **3 minutes.**

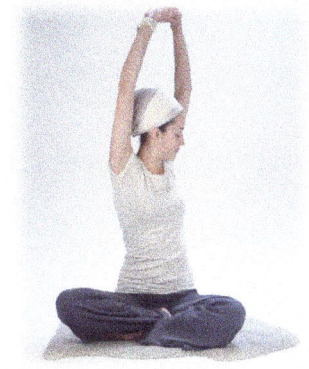

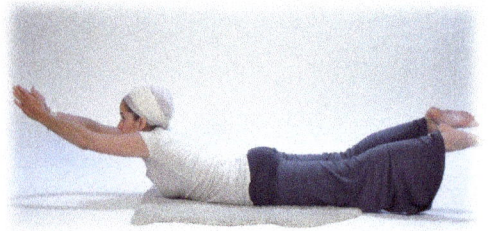

4. Lie on stomach with arms stretched out in front, palms together. Lift head, hands and feet as high as possible. BOF for **3 minutes**.

Lie on stomach with hands back by hips and relax for **1 minute**.

5. On stomach reach back, hold ankles, arch up into Bow Pose with BOF, and rock back and forth on stomach for **2 minutes**.

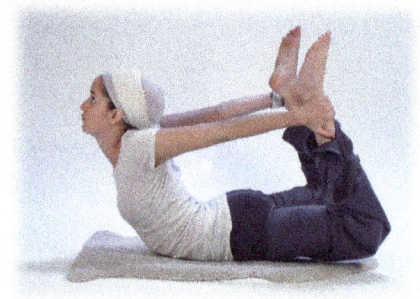

Relax on stomach for **1 minute**.

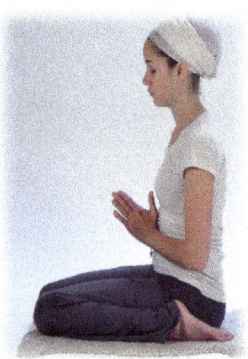

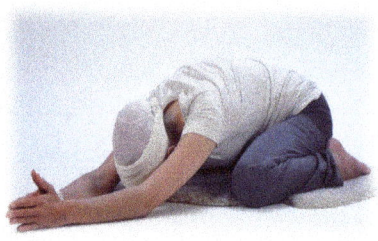

6. Sit on the heels and drop into Celibate Pose with hips down on the ground. Put hands in Prayer Pose at navel point and inhale. Exhale and bend forward with arms stretched out in front, hands still in Prayer Pose and place forehead on floor. Continue to inhale up and exhale down for **5 minutes**.

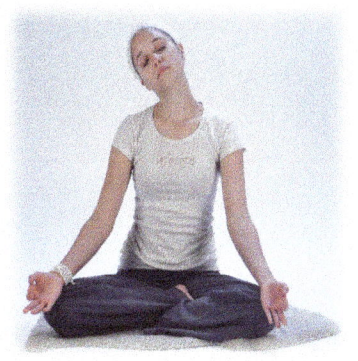

7. Easy Pose, hands in GM on the knees. Roll the head in large circles from left to right for **1½ minutes**.

Switch directions; roll the head from right to left for **1½ minutes**.

8. Easy Pose, hands on knees.

Roll shoulders from front to the back for **1 ½ minutes.**

Reverse direction and roll shoulders from the back to the front for **1 ½ minutes.**

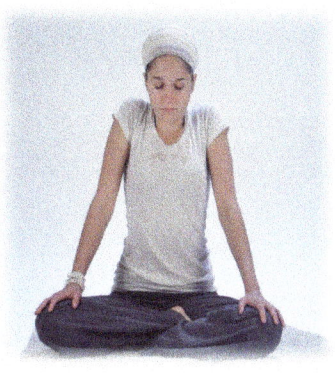

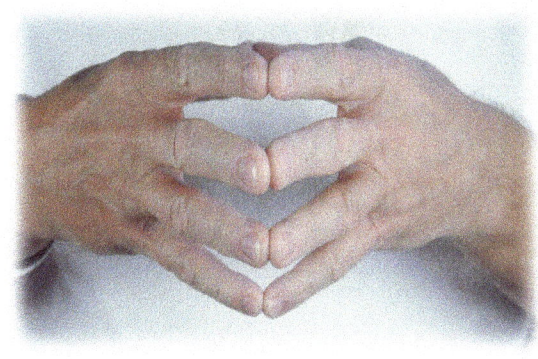

9. Easy Pose with hands in Prayer Pose at heart chakra. Spread palms apart so only tips of fingers touch; thumbs point at the heart two inches from the body. Spread fingers wide apart pointing away from the body. Inhale through nose in one breath, and then forcibly exhale through puckered mouth in eight strokes. Continue for **11 minutes**.

10. Long Deep Relaxation

Meditation To Create Your Destiny
Harmonize the 4th Body

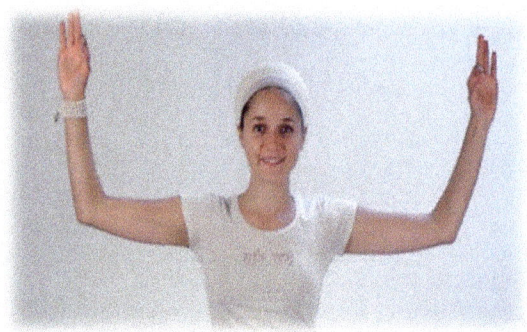

Part 1) Easy Pose with arms up and bent 90º at elbow with forearms perpendicular to the ground and fingers pointing up. Hands in GM, palms face away from body.

Close the eyes. In a monotone chant the mantra,
'*Waho, Waho, Waho, Waho, Guru, Guru, Guru, Guru.*'

Meditate at the heart for **11 to 31 minutes.**

Part 2) Sit in the same posture.

Inhale in 4 strokes, mentally repeat the mantra:
'*Waho, Waho, Waho, Waho.*'

Exhale in 4 strokes, mentally repeat the mantra:
'*Guru, Guru, Guru, Guru.*'

Repeat for **11 to 31 minutes.**

To End) Sing the Long Time Sun song.

This meditation brings neutrality and lightness, and makes large problems seem small.

Fifth Body
Physical Body
Kundalini Yoga to Create Your Destiny
Harmonize the 5th Body
Balance the Heart and Small Intestine Meridians

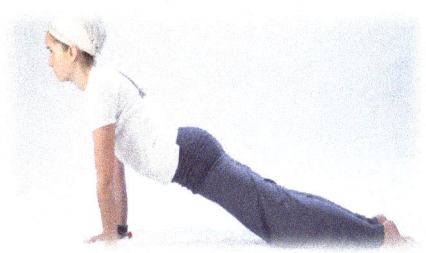

1. Platform Pose: Inhale up in Platform Pose, keep head in line with the body, apply MB and exhale down. Continue to inhale up and exhale down for **1-2 minutes.**

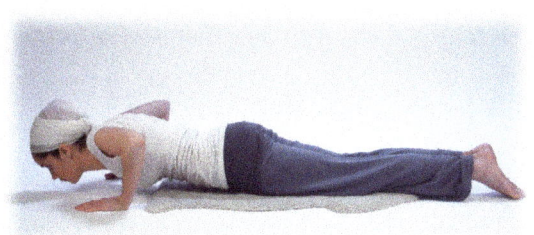

2. Repeat asana and reverse the breath. Inhale down, apply MB and exhale in Platform Pose. Continue for **1-2 minutes.**

3. Repeat **3 cycles.**

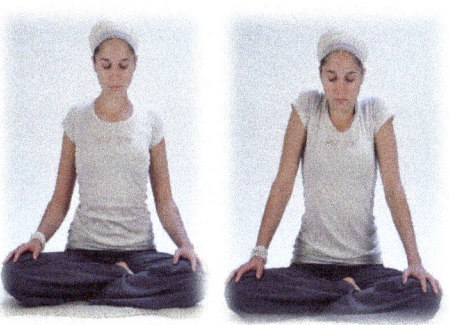

4. Inhale, pull both shoulders up and exhale, release shoulders down. Continue for **2 minutes.**

5. Easy Pose, roll head to the right for **1 minute**, then roll head to the left for **1 minute**.

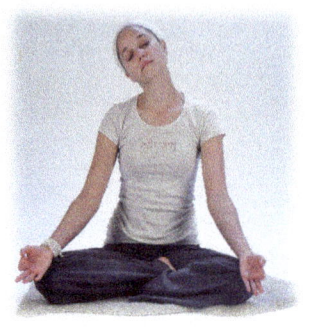

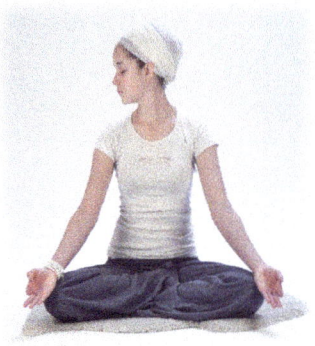 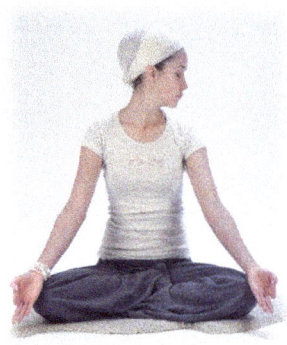

6. Easy Pose, hands in GM. Inhale, turn the head to the left and say '*Wha*.' Turn the head to the middle and say '*He*', turn the head to the right and say '*Guru*'. Repeat for **3-11 minutes.**

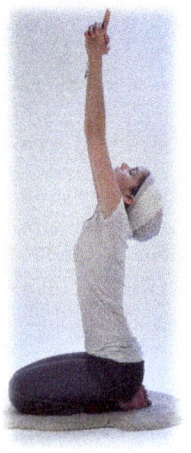 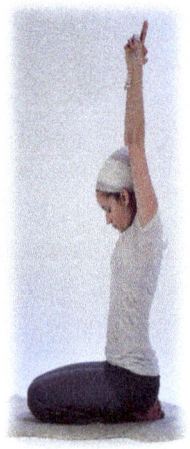

7. On heels, arms up in Sat Kriya position. Engage slight neck lock, inhale and drop head backward. Exhale and bring chin to chest. Continue this motion for **3 minutes.**

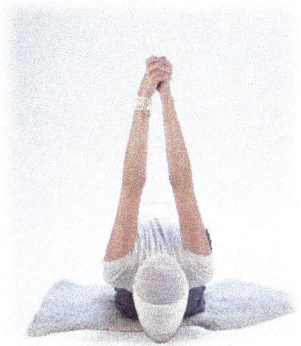

8. Sit on heels, interlace fingers behind back, bring forehead to ground and raise arms up into Yoga Mudra. Hold for **3 minutes.**

9. Long Deep Relaxation

Meditation To Create Your Destiny
Harmonize the 5th Body

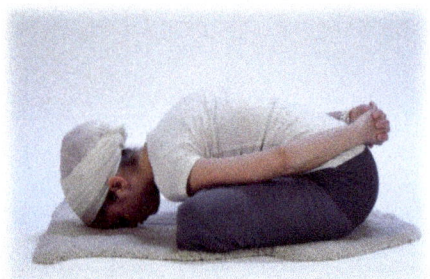

Part 1) Easy Pose with hands in VL on back at the base of the spine. In this sitting posture chant the mantra *'Hum'* vibrating the sound in the back of the throat. Chant *'Har'* and put the forehead on the ground. Continue this meditative movement for **5-11 minutes.**

Part 2) Easy Pose, hands in VL in lap. Concentrate at the third eye. Chant *'Hari Har'* in three separate tongue movements: *'Har-i-Har'*, touch the soft palate with tip of the tongue on both the *'Har'* sounds.

Concentrate with entire consciousness on this triple tongue movement. Continue for **5-11 minutes.**

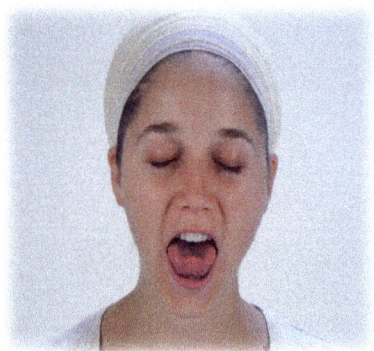

Part 3) Stick tongue out, don't let any saliva touch the tongue, and breathe through open mouth. Continue for **2 minutes**.

To End) Sing the Long Time Sun song.

Sixth Body
The Arc Line

Kundalini Yoga to Create Your Destiny
Harmonize the 6th Body
Balance the Pericardium and Triple Warmer Meridians

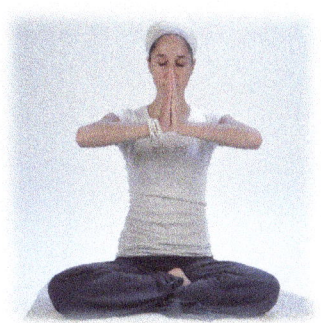

1. Easy Pose with hands in GM on knees. Focus at third eye. Inhale, mentally vibrate *'Sat'*, exhale, and mentally vibrate *'Nam'* **for 3 minutes.**

2. Easy Pose, bring palms together at nose level, keep the elbows level with shoulders. Have maximum pressure on the hands with LDB. Hold for **3 minutes.**

Sit with hands in the lap for **1 minute.**

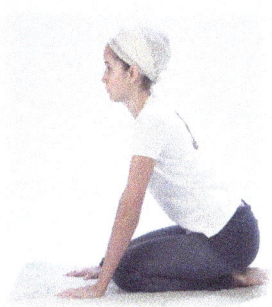
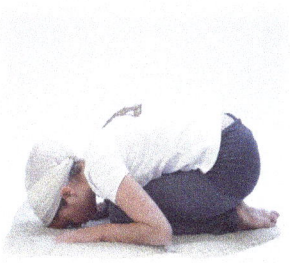

3. On the heels with hands out in front of you on the floor. Vibrate the sound *'Sat'* in the up position and then vibrate the sound *'Nam'* in the down position as you bring forehead to the ground. Continue for **15 minutes.**

Easy Pose with hands in lap for **1 minute.**

4. Easy Pose with palms together at heart chakra about 1 inch above the sternum. Mentally vibrate peace and love for the entire universe and hold this intention. LDB for **3 minutes.**

5. Sit on heels and stretch the right leg out straight in front. Lean over and hold the right big toe with both hands. Continue with LDB **for 3 minutes.** Inhale, then exhale and hold the breath out for **8 seconds** and apply MB.

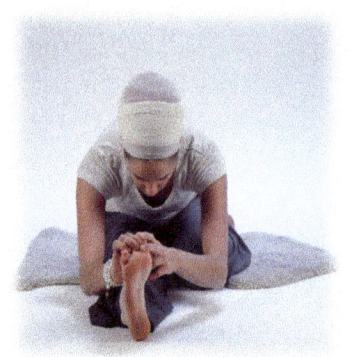

Change sides and repeat the asana with left leg out straight.

Relax in Easy Pose with the hands in the lap for **1 minute**

Meditation To Create Your Destiny
Harmonize the 6th Body

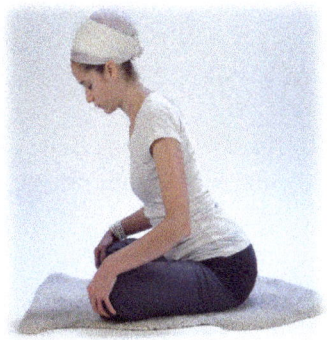 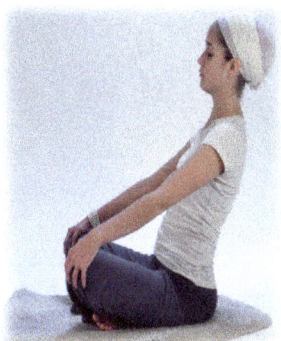

Part 1) Easy Pose and concentrate at third eye. Hands hold on to kneecaps. Chant '*Sat*' and lean forward 60°. Keep spine straight and chant '*Nam*' and lean backward 60°. Continue for **11-31 minutes.**

Note: The spine is straight throughout and the buttocks stay stationary as the head and upper body move forward and back.

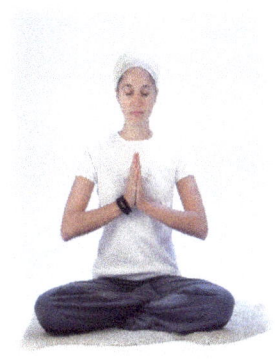

Part 2) Easy Pose with hands together at center of the chest in Prayer Pose. Inhale, then chant '*SaaAAAaa*' on the exhale. Start with a low volume then increase the volume in the middle and then decrease the volume for the last 1/3 of the chant. Continue for **3 minutes.**

Part 3) Easy Pose with hands together at the center of the chest in Prayer Pose. Inhale, then chant the mantra '*Sa*' six times in a monotone on the exhale.

Continue for **3 minutes.**

To End) Sing the Long Time Sun song.

The Seventh Body
The Aura

Kundalini Yoga to Harmonize the 7th Body

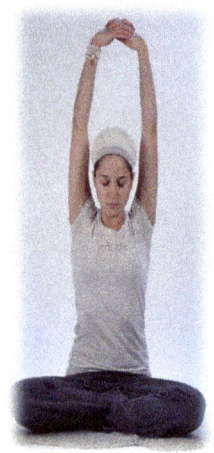

1. Easy Pose with hands above the head in VL. Pull the hands apart with LDB for **3 minutes**.

Inhale, apply MB and hold for **20 seconds**. Exhale, apply MB and hold out for the count of eight.

Hands in GM on the knees with LDB. Concentrate on the tip of the nose for **5 minutes**.

2. Hands in VL above the head. Extend the thumbs out and put pressure on the thumbs.

LDB and try to pull the hands apart for **3 minutes**.

Inhale, hold the breath and apply MB for **20 seconds,** then exhale, apply MB and hold the breath out for **8 seconds**.

Inhale, and lower the hands down into GM on the knees. Focus at the tip of the nose with LDB for **3 minutes**.

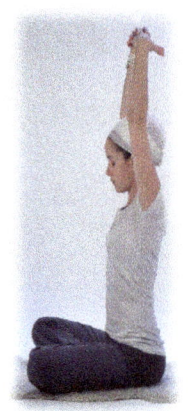

3. Hands above the head in VL. Extend forefingers up and press them together while also pulling apart on the VL. Continue for 3 minutes. Inhale, apply MB, and hold for 20 seconds. Exhale, apply MB and hold out for the count of eight. Inhale, exhale and lower the hands into GM on the knees with LDB and focus at the tip of the nose for **3 minutes**.

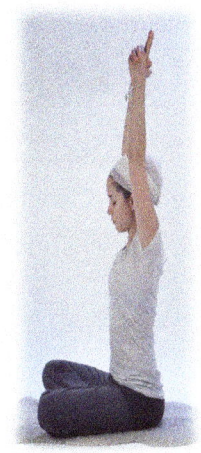

4. Easy Pose with the arms extended straight up and spread out 60° with the fingers spread wide apart. Concentrate on creating a funnel from the hands leading into the top of the head at the 10th gate. BOF for **3 minutes**.

5. Easy Pose with hands in GM. Meditate on energy flowing out the top of the head; visualize expanding into your protective aura. Continue for **3 minutes**.

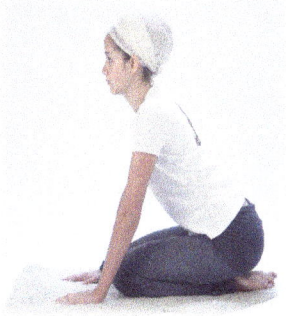 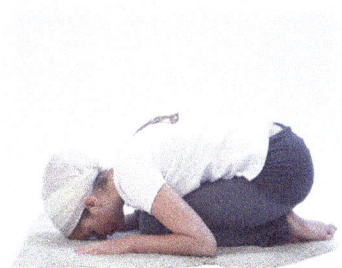

6. Sit in Celibate Pose, or on the heels. Put your palms on the ground in front of the knees. Inhale with the arms straight and mentally vibrate '*Sat*'. Exhale as you bring your forehead to the ground and mentally vibrate '*Nam*'. Continue for **3 minutes**.

7. Sit on heels and place the forehead on the ground in Gurpranam. Continue for **3 minutes**.

8. Long Deep Relaxation

Meditation To Create Your Destiny
Harmonize the 7th Body

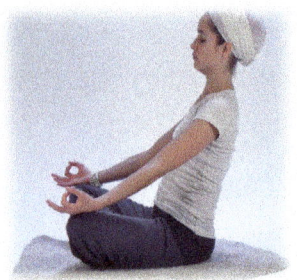

Part 1) Easy Pose with hands in GM on the knees. Lean the body back 60° with neck in alignment with the spine. Concentrate at the center of the skull and hold this position with LDB for **3 minutes**.

Part 2) Sit in Rock Pose with hands in VL in the lap. Lean body back 60° and concentrate at the top of the head with LDB for **3 minutes**. Inhale as you sit up straight, and hold the breath. Concentrate at the top of the head.

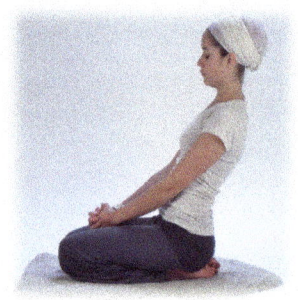

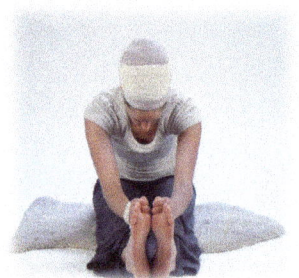

Part 3) Sit with legs straight out in front, hold the toes, release the belly forward to the thighs with LDB for **3 minutes**.

Part 4) Sit with legs stretched out in front, press toes forward. Place the hands on thighs and lean back 60°. Apply neck lock. Concentrate internally and look into the top of the head. Continue the meditation for **11 minutes**, then inhale and gather the energy at the top of the head.

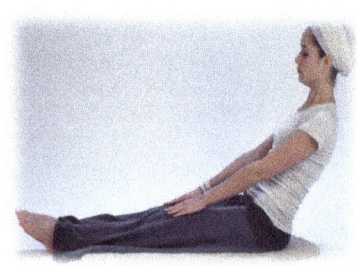

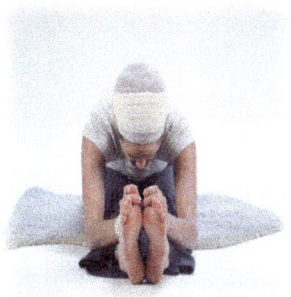

Part 5) Sit with legs out in front, release into a forward stretch with LDB for **3 minutes.**

Part 6) Sit in Rock Pose on heels and focus on the back of the head opposite from the third eye point with LDB for **3 minutes.**

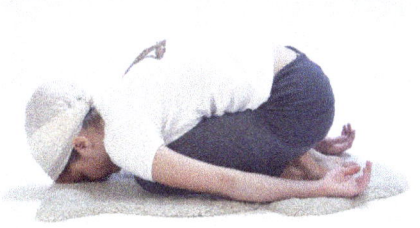

Part 7) Bend forward, place forehead on the ground and relax for **5 minutes.**

To End) Sing the Long Time Sun song.

Eighth Body
Pranic Body

Kundalini Yoga to Create Your Destiny
Harmonize the 8th Body

1. Easy Pose and raise both arms up to 60°, palms face up with LDB. Hold for **3 minutes.**

2. Easy Pose with arms in Sat Kriya position and BOF for **3 minutes.**

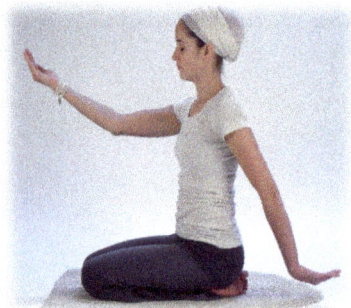

3. Sit on heels, extend the right-arm in front of you with the palm up, elbow slightly bent, hand cupped and extend the left arm out behind you, elbow bent, hand cupped with LDB. Continue for **1 minute**, then:
   Rest **30 seconds**
   Repeat asana for **1 minute**
   Rest **30 seconds**
   Repeat asana for **1 minute**
   Rest for **30 seconds**

4. Easy Pose and do neck rolls to the left for **1 minute** then switch directions and continue for **another minute.**

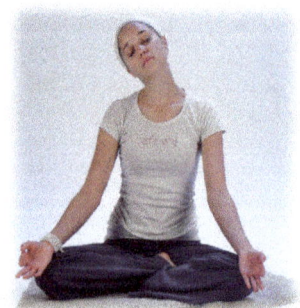

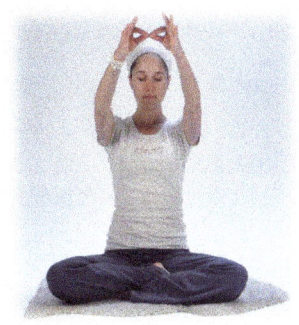

5. Easy Pose, hands in GM, palms face each other and thumb tips touch. Raise the arms up 60º in front. BOF for **3 minutes**.

6. Yogi walk, **50 repetitions.** Remain up on the toes, with the hands in GM, arms out to the sides, elbows bent and forearms up perpendicular to the ground. Powerfully inhale as one knee comes up and exhale down, then repeat on other side.

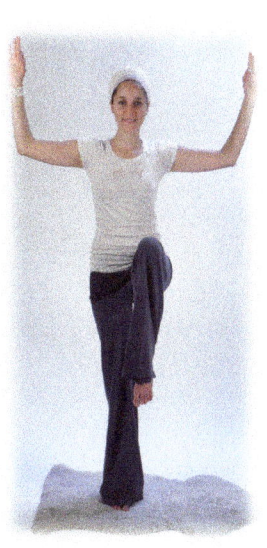

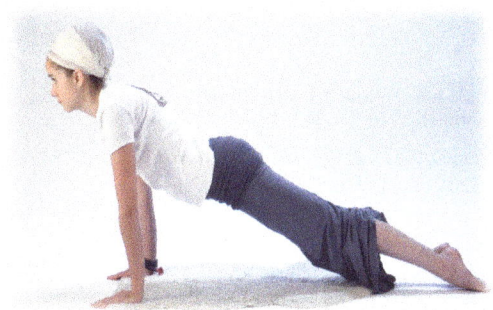

7. Lay on stomach with hands underneath your shoulders, spread the fingers wide. Raise the body totally straight into Front Platform Pose up on your hands and tops of the feet and apply neck lock. Continue for **1-3 minutes**. Inhale and exhale and lie on stomach, turn head to one side, arms back by sides, palms face up. Relax for **1 minute.**

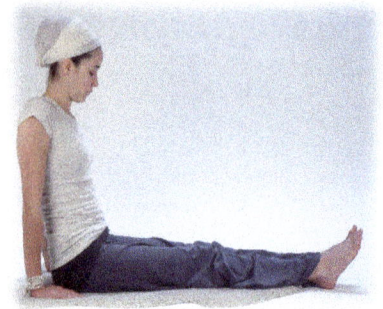

8. Sit up with legs extended straight out in front, hands down on the ground by the hips. Inhale and lift the buttocks off the ground. Exhale and drop the buttocks to the ground. Continue body drops **26 times**.

9. Easy Pose with hands in a modified Prayer Pose with only the fingertips touching in front of the heart center. Point the thumbs back toward the heart and point the fingers away from the heart with BOF. Continue for **3 minutes** with LDB.

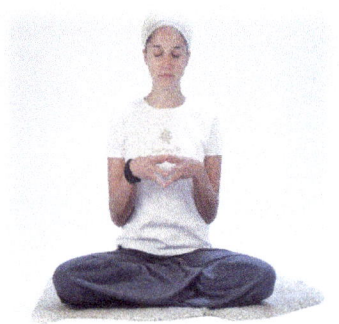

10. Long Deep Relaxation

Meditation To Create Your Destiny
Harmonize the 8th Body

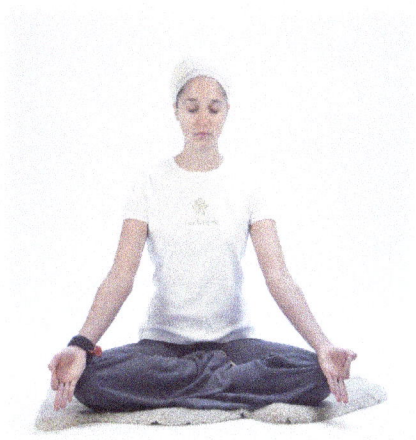

Part 1) Easy Pose with hands in GM on knees. Inhale in four parts and visualize white light coming in through the crown chakra. Exhale slowly in one long breath and visualize a blue light, like a gas flame, emanating from each of your pores and filling your aura. Continue for **5-15 minutes.**

Lie down in Corpse Pose and rest for **3 minutes.**

2. Repeat the meditation and increase the inhale from 4 to 9 parts. Continue for **5-15 minutes.**

Relax in Corpse Pose for **3 minutes.**

This kriya will produce a lot of psychic heat, which creates deep clearing

Ninth Body
Subtle Body

Kundalini Yoga to Create Your Destiny
Harmonize the 9th Body

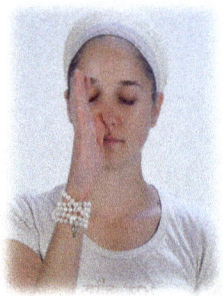 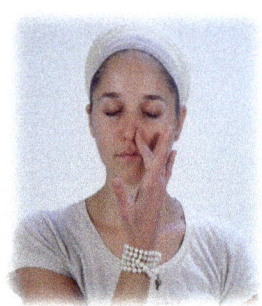

1. Easy Pose with the thumb blocking the right nostril. Inhale through the left nostril, then block the left nostril with the middle finger of the right hand, release the right thumb and exhale through the right nostril. Then inhale right and exhale left. Then inhale left and exhale right. Continue alternating nostril pranayam for **3 minutes.**

2. Easy Pose with arms up at 60° with palms flat as if holding up the sky. LDB and concentrate on the warmth in palms and fingers for **3 minutes.**

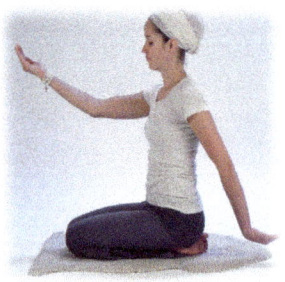

3. Easy Pose with right arm extended out in front parallel to the earth with elbow slightly bent and hand cupped. Extend the left arm out behind with elbow slightly bent and hand cupped. Both palms face up. On the inhale, feel the energy move from the hands to the heart. On the exhale, feel the energy move from the heart to the eyes and to the hands. Continue this breath visualization with LDB for **1 minute.**

Change sides and continue for **1 minute.** After **1 minute** changes sides again and finally, after **1 minute** change sides again (for a total of **4 minutes.**)

4. On knees and elbows, sides of hands touch and form a cup in front of face. Stare into palms. Touch the feet together and raise them off the floor. Hold with LDB for **5 to 7 minutes.**

Relax on stomach for **3 minutes.**

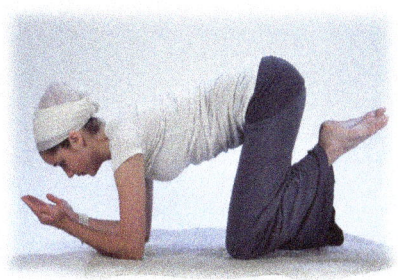

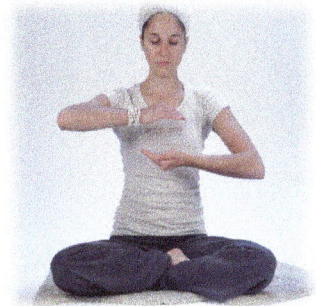

5. Easy Pose with both palms at solar plexus as if holding a ball. Left palm faces up and right palm faces down. The hands are 5 inches apart and 1 inch from the body. Focus at solar plexus and feel a ball of energy between the palms. Feel the pranic heat and focus with LDB for **7 minutes.**

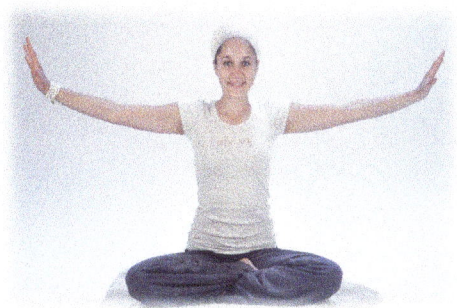

6. Easy Pose with the arms stretched out to the sides parallel to the earth. Palms face outward as if holding up the walls.

Inhale hold the breath and bring the hands 4 inches apart at the heart center then move them to ¼ -inch apart then back out to 4 inches apart.

Repeat this pumping movement **8 times**

Then exhale and move the arms back to original position out to sides.

Inhale and repeat the pumping movement **8 times** while holding the breath and continue for **7 minutes.**

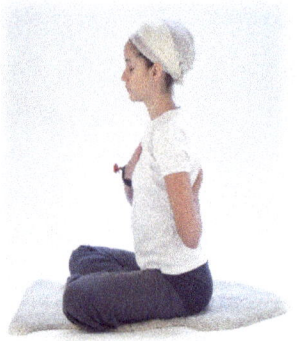 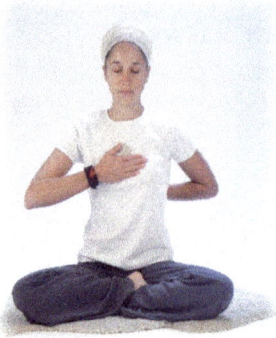

7. Easy Pose, place right palm on heart center and left palm facing out on the back at heart center. Chant '*Ek ong kara, sata nama, siri whaa hay guru*' for **7 minutes.**

8. Long Deep Relaxation

Meditation To Create Your Destiny
Harmonize the 9th Body

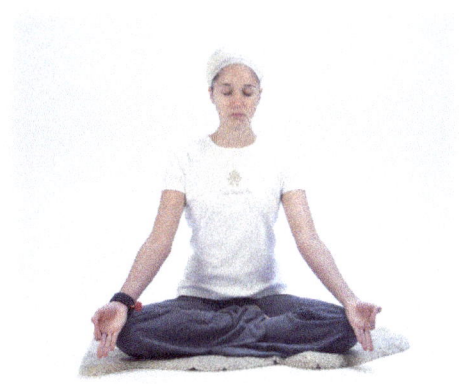

Easy Pose, hands in GM on knees.
Apply slight MB during entire meditation.

8 part segmented inhale and one long exhale:

On each of the 8 inhales, internally vibrate '*Wahe*' as you connect to each of the 8 chakras and project a light around the body.

Exhale with one long deep breath and mentally vibrate '*Guru*' and release all to infinity.

Practice this meditation for **11-31 minutes** or **up to 2 ½ hours.**

This meditation heals, consoles, and washes away all constraints.

To End) Sing the Long Time Sun song.

Tenth Body
Radiant Body

Kundalini Yoga to Create Your Destiny
Harmonize the 10th Body

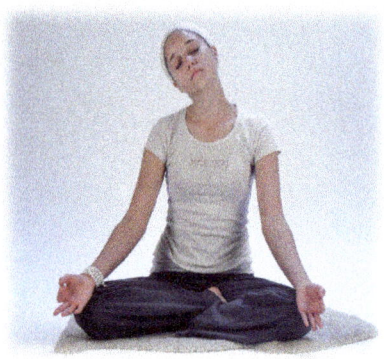

1. Easy Pose and roll neck to the left, continue for one minute. Switch directions and roll neck to right for **one minute.**

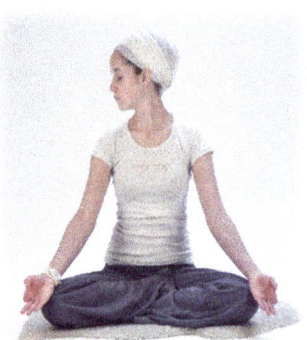
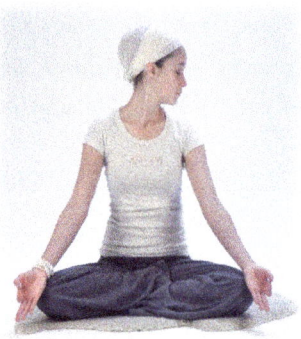

2. Easy Pose hands in GM (continued next page)
Turn head to the left and say the mantra '*Wha*'.
Turn to the center say the mantra ' *hay*'.
Turn to the right say the mantra '*Guru*'.
Continue for **11 minutes.**

Rest with hands in lap for **1 minute.**

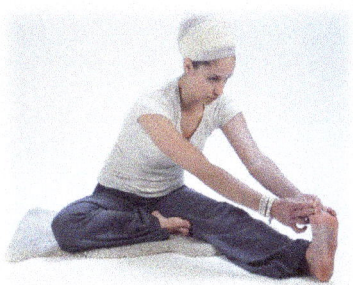

3. Sit with left leg out in front. Tuck the right foot into pelvic area. Reach down and hold the big toe of left foot with both index fingers and press the tip of the toe with both thumbs. Pull spine straight and stare at the big toe of the left foot. Inhale, then exhale the breath and apply MB and hold for **8 seconds**. Inhale, then exhale, apply MB and hold for **8 seconds**. Continue for **7 ½ minutes**. Switch sides and repeat with the right leg out.

Relax in Corpse Pose for **5 minutes**.

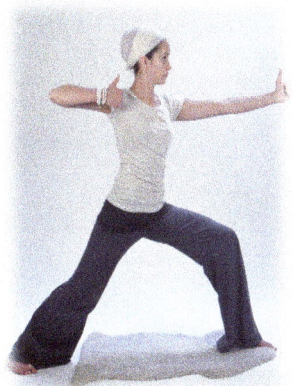

4. Archer Pose with left foot forward and the right leg back. The left arm is up in front of the body with hand in fist and the thumb raised up. The right hand is bent at the elbow as if you are pulling back on a bowstring. Concentrate over the tip of the left thumb with BOF **for 5 ½ minutes**. Switch sides and hold Archer Pose with right leg forward **for 5 ½ minutes**.

5. Long Deep Relaxation

Meditation To Create Your Destiny
Harmonize the 10th Body

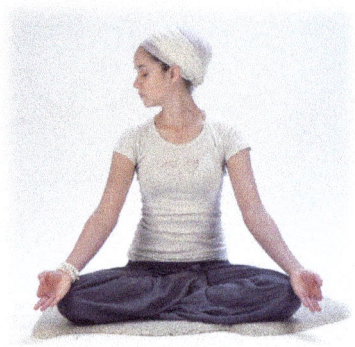

Part 1) Easy Pose, concentrate at root of nose and allow for pressure to build up. Inhale in a three-part segmented breath, and mentally repeat '*Sat Nam*' on each segment of the breath. Head remains still.
Exhale with a three-part segmented breath out.

The head turns on the exhale:
  1/3 exhale, turn head to the left and mentally vibrate '*Wa.*'
  1/3 exhale, return head straight and mentally vibrate '*Hay.*'
  1/3 exhale, turn head to right and mentally vibrate '*Guru.*'

Continue for **7 minutes**. At end of meditation: Feel the prana that was generated, and experience the positive energy from all planets in the universe supporting you as a being of light.

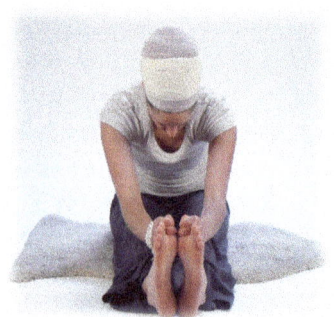

Part 2) Sit with the legs stretched out in front. Hold big toes, relax into forward bend, and relax shoulders. Focus on third eye and bathe the brain in prana and light. Maintain for **3 minutes.**

Part 3) Repeat part 1.

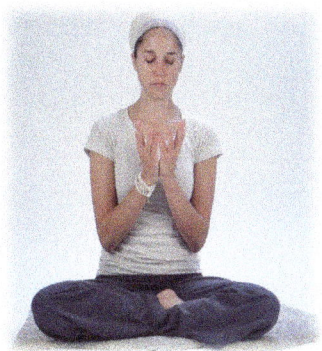

Part 4) Easy Pose. Hands in Lotus Mudra, 6 inches in front of heart center. Sides of hands touch; relax fingers and thumbs and form a lotus flower.

Drishti (eye focus): 1/10th open and stare past the tip of the nose at the thumbs. LDB and feel hands fill with fire.

Eleventh Embodiment

Kundalini Yoga to Create Your Destiny
Harmonize the 11th Body

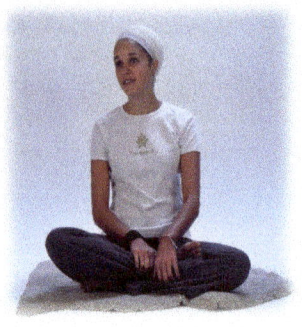

Part 1) Easy Pose and hold shins. Spine Flex: Inhale and pull the spine forward, exhale and relax the spine back. Do this for **3 minutes**.

Relax hands in lap, LDB for **1 minute**.

2. Rock Pose. Spine flex with the hands on the thighs for **3 minutes**.

Rest hands in lap for **1 minute**.

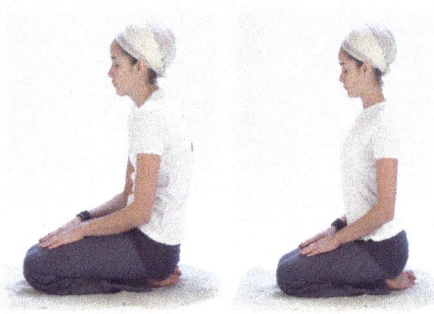

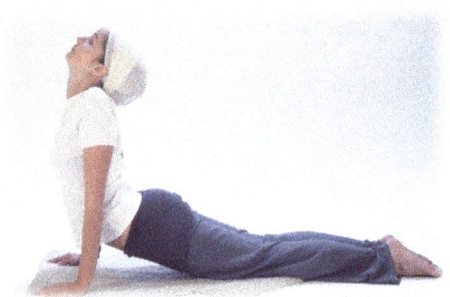

3. Lie on stomach, hands underneath the shoulders and lift up into Cobra Pose. Inhale through the nose and exhale through the open mouth with the teeth clenched for **3 minutes**.

Inhale, hold breath, apply MB and hold for **10 seconds**. Lower down; turn head to one side with arms by sides and palms up. Relax for **1 minute**.

4. Up on knees and hands for Cat Cow. Inhale, stretch head up and spine down, then exhale and move head down and spine up.

Continue at a fast pace for **3 minutes.**

Inhale and hold with MB for **20 seconds** then exhale and sit back.

Rest with hands in lap for **1 minute.**

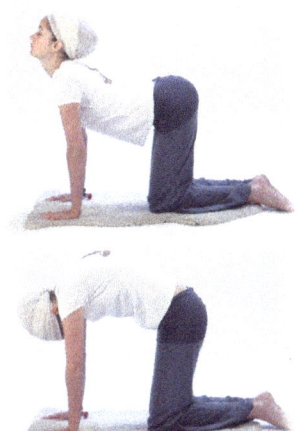

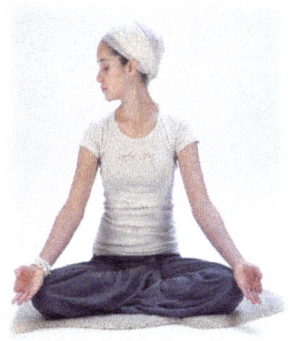 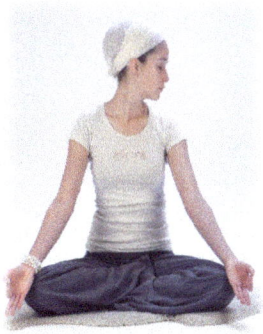

5. Easy Pose hands in GM. Inhale and turn the head over left shoulder. Exhale, turning the head to the right shoulder. Continue for **1 minute.**

Reverse the pranayam: Inhale, turn head over right shoulder then exhale, turning head over left shoulder.

Rest with hands in lap for **1 minute.**

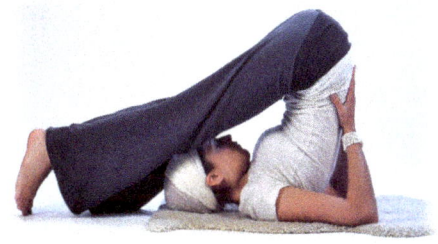

6. Lie on the back, and bring feet over head into Plow Pose with LDB for **3 minutes**. At the end, slowly lower down vertebra by vertebra, then relax on back for **1 minute.**

7. On back, bring knees to chest, wrap arms around knees, then roll back and forth on spine. Inhale up and exhale down for **3 minutes.** Rest on back for **1 minute.**

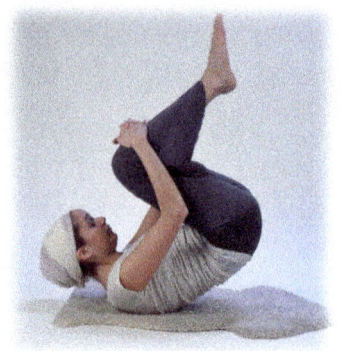

8. Sit on heels, with hands above head for Sat Kriya. Do Sat Kriya for **3 minutes.**

Long Deep Relaxation for **11 minutes.**

Meditation To Create Your Destiny
Harmonize the 11th Body

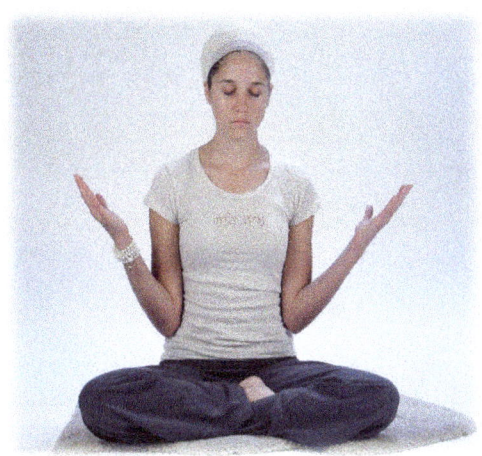

Easy Pose, elbows by sides with hands up at 60° with the palms open. Vibrate "Sat Nam" as you make fists with both hands with the thumbs outside of the fist. Then release "*Wahe Guru* " and open hands releasing all thoughts to the universe. Continue the hand movement and:

> Chant mantra out loud for **5 minutes**.
> Whisper mantra for **5 minutes**.
> Internally repeat the mantra for **10 minutes**.
> Whisper mantra for **5 minutes**.
> Chant mantra out loud for **5 minutes**.

To End) Sing the Long Time Sun song.

This meditation 'massages' the brain and gives a person total control and mastery of all ten bodies.

About the Authors

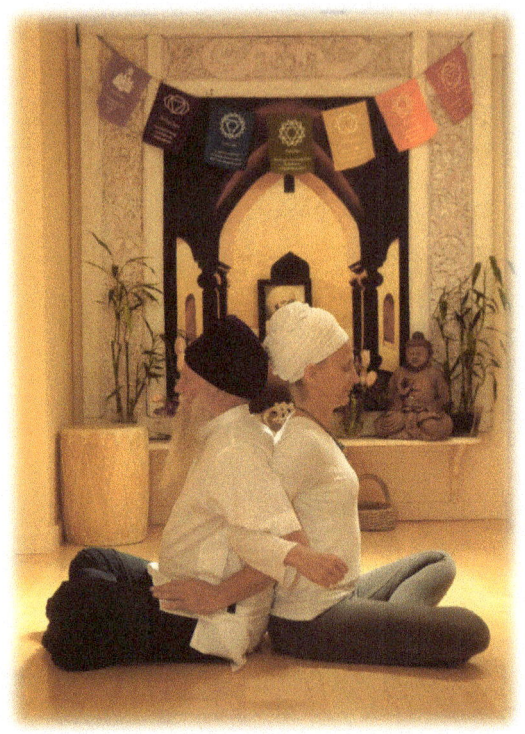

Dr. Guruchander was born and raised in Texas. He received his BA in Business Administration from Southern Methodist University in 1972, and his Doctor of Chiropractic degree from Pasadena College of Chiropractic in Pasadena, California, in 1982.

Dr Guruchander began studying yoga with Yogi Bhajan in 1972, and became his personal chiropractor in 1985. In addition to his training in chiropractic, he has studied many forms of Oriental healing. He is the director of GRD Health Clinic in Santa Fe, New Mexico, which offers chiropractic, acupuncture, massage therapy, and other natural healing therapies.

Kirn was born and raised in the Netherlands, Europe. She moved to the USA in 1975 when she was 15, and was introduced to Kundalini Yoga. This powerful practice awakened her life-long passion for the expression of Purest Potential. She began assisting in the production of many women and children's educational and training programs under the direct supervision of Yogi Bhajan.

She has created an energy healing modality, "Yogic Energy Healing" which uses radionics, radiesthesia and yoga to increase awareness about physical, mental and spiritual wellness. Her current work focuses on integrating the teachings of kundalini yoga, prosperity, energy healing, and yoga: all for the expression of Purest Potential.

Kirn and Guruchander serve as directors for the non-profit yoga center Purest Potential; located at 1505 Llano Street in Santa Fe, NM; the only yoga center in Santa Fe dedicated to teachings of kundalini yoga. Both Guruchander and Kirn are KRI certified teacher trainers for all 3 levels of kundalini yoga and travel extensively throughout the world sharing these beautiful teachings.

They are the owners of Purest Potential, a company that **shares techniques so you can design a life which supports your purpose.**

Kirn, Guruchander and their 2 children, Gurumittar and Gurusundesh, enjoy a life of enchantment in Santa Fe, NM.

Kirn and Guruchander have also authored *Tantric Numerology* and *Purest Potential – A Yogi's guide to brilliance*, which, together with this book, comprise a healing trilogy for those in search of sustainable enlightenment, sovereignty and prosperity.

With Love and Light

Sat Nam

For support and inspiration on this journey to manifest Purest Potential we invite you to our website www.purestpotential.com.

www.ingramcontent.com/pod-product-compliance
Lightning Source LLC
Chambersburg PA
CBHW051549010526
44118CB00022B/2633